The End of Sex

The Gender Revolution and its Consequences

Stephen Whitehead

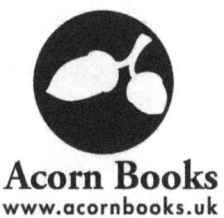

Acorn Books
www.acornbooks.uk

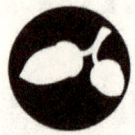

Published in 2025 by
Acorn Books
An Imprint of
Andrews UK Limited
West Wing Studios
Unit 166, The Mall
Luton, LU1 2TL

Copyright © 2025
Stephen Whitehead

The right of
Stephen Whitehead to be
identified as author of this work
has been asserted in accordance with
the Copyright, Designs and Patents Act 1988.

All rights reserved. No reproduction, copy or transmission of this publication may be made without express prior written permission. No paragraph of this publication may be reproduced, copied or transmitted except with express prior written permission or in accordance with the provisions of the Copyright Act 1956 (as amended). Any person who commits any unauthorised act in relation to this publication may be liable to criminal prosecution and civil claims for damage.

The views and opinions expressed herein belong to the authors and do not necessarily reflect those of Acorn Books or Andrews UK Limited.

Contents

About the Author iv

Praise for The End of Sex v

Acknowledgements viii

Foreword x

Chapter 1: The Gender Revolution 1

Chapter 2: Reflections on the Rise of Feminism: 1950 to 1990 20

Chapter 3: Independent Femininity 42

Chapter 4: Men's Responses 78

Chapter 5: Living Apart, Growing Apart 116

Chapter 6: The End of Sex 157

Afterword 184

About the Author

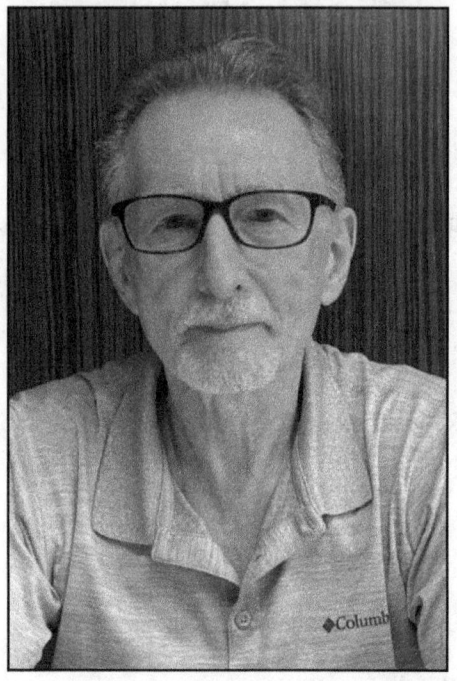

Dr Stephen Whitehead is a British sociologist, feminist, writer, and internationally recognised expert in gender studies, men and masculinities, femininities, identity, and education. He is known for his progressive approach to issues of identity, gender, inclusivity and organisational culture. He has created and helped develop numerous concepts notably:

- Total Inclusivity
- Totally Inclusive Self-Love
- Hegemonic Masculinity
- Toxic Masculinity
- Hegemonic Femininity
- Independent Femininity
- Toxic Femininity

Since 1999, he has published twenty academic and mainstream books, covering topics such as gender, masculinities, identity, self-love, globalization, education and organisations. Stephen has lived in Thailand since 2009.

www.stephen-whitehead.com

Praise for The End of Sex

A thought-provoking and ambitious work that captures the global scale and urgency of the gender divergence we are seeing today. The themes of rising independent femininity, the crisis of traditional masculinity, and the impact of technology on relationships are all extremely timely, and in many ways, unsettling.

Caroline Codsi,
Founder, Women in Governance & Parity Certification,
Montreal, Canada

A strong, powerful, enlightening, and very timely book, written with authority and a definite sense of urgency. This book deserves to be read by anyone concerned at the current state of gender relationships.

Dr Denry Machin,
Educational Consultant and Author,
Bangkok, Thailand

Dr Stephen Whitehead's new book is an insightful, bold and creative exploration that challenges the foundations of gender and sexuality. Stephen's imaginative interpretations of the social, geopolitical interweaved with personal narratives offer readers an opportunity to understand at an affective level their relationship between the personal and the social. A timely contribution to the ongoing debate about the future of men, women, sex and gender and much more in a rapidly changing world.

Dr Roy Moodley,
Professor of Psychology,
University of Toronto, Canada.

Stephen Whitehead has produced a powerful and necessary book – insightful, timely, and thought-provoking. The writing flows with clarity and purpose, and the depth of analysis reveals a rare understanding of the complexities of gender and intimacy in our time. This is more than just a book; it is a conversation starter, a mirror, and an invitation to reflect. It is bound to resonate widely and leave a lasting impression.

Constanza Fernández Arce,
Author and Educationalist,
Santiago, Chile

The End of Sex provides a provocative and clear-eyed reflection and insight into how AI will intersect with men's evolving (and often troubled) sense of identity in this era of gender divergence. Stephen Whitehead's analysis of how some men – particularly those alienated by feminist progress and/or shaped by toxic masculinity – will seek out AI not as a partner but as a proxy, is both accurate and timely.

James Edward L. Lara,
Founder, Nova-Lila AI Initiative,
Tokyo, Japan

The End of Sex is a wise, compassionate and discerning critique of the politics of gender identity. Expertly drawing from feminist scholarship, Stephen interrogates male fundamentalism and power in the era of Trump and Tate, challenging toxic masculinity and the incorrigible constructs of the gender binary. This is a profoundly ethical book. It doesn't shy away from the scale of the task, but it also offers hope and ways forward, especially for those working in progressive education and equality, diversity and inclusion (EDI) initiatives.

Dr Francis Farrell,
Senior Lecturer in Education,
Edge Hill University, UK.

There's something in and, increasingly, on the air. The news is still full of accounts of misogyny, violence and injustice delivered by men and borne by women. But it also contains accounts of resistance, countervailing words and actions, and progressive movements in which women gather themselves, and show self-regard and dignity, authority and autonomy. T'was ever thus – well, maybe. This book returns to possibilities that Isadora Wing could only have dreamed about.

This book takes us on a journey through gender relations during Stephen Whitehead's lifetime and into the future. The long view back that he traces is carefully-drawn, explaining how feminist thought and femininities and the responses that have articulated masculinities have developed. But it's not a dry or shrill history. His own experience and that of his family, as much as on events familiar from the news and stats from the world over, are deftly woven and carry his account of the changing pattern of relations between women and men, and the arguments that made a difference.

In moving from analysing the past and present to speculating about future change, he points to one, intimately-connected touchstone of gender relations – sex. Technologies like the condom and the pill revolutionised sex (and gender) relations. The final Chapter of the book offers some provocative thoughts on how emerging technologies might offer women ways to escape, still further, the assumed 'entitlements' of men (writ as the necessary condition of humanity). As Stephen Whitehead puts it: "The one standout question which each straight woman will have to ask herself is; which do I love more, men or independence?" As we wait for his 'AI de Beauvoir' to respond, we have at least this book, accessible, persuasive, and profound.

Dr Steve Cropper,
Emeritus Professor of Management,
Keele University, UK.

Acknowledgements

A great many individuals have, over the decades, made vital contributions to my understanding of gender and its relationship to identity, masculinities, and power: I thank all of them. Three who were pivotal to my intellectual development from the early nineties were Professor Sheila Scraton, Professor Jeff Hearn and Professor David Morgan. I am especially grateful to those who read drafts of this book and subsequently provided immensely useful feedback; Caroline Codsi, Denry Machin, Steve Cropper, Roy Moodley, Constanza Fernández Arce, James Edward L. Lara and Francis Farrell. Also, my thanks to Sara Ellingham and Amanda Field of AUK.

For Gavin, Jay, Robert, Eleanor and Dia

Foreword

Shortly after completing this book in January 2025, several events occurred confirming its hypothesis, which is that a global gender revolution is leading to dramatic changes in the lives of women and men around the world; changes which quite obviously are not going to go unchallenged by social conservatives, male fundamentalists and the like. The first two events happened simultaneously: newly re-elected US President Donald Trump instigating his formal kickback against the gender revolution by introducing policies designed explicitly to eliminate DEI (Diversity, Equity and Inclusion) rules and initiatives across the public and private sectors; and Elon Musk, the world's wealthiest person, finally entering the realm of politics alongside Trump and with the same intent, that is to 'Make America Great Again' by "ensuring competent white men are in charge".[1]

While this curtailment of DEI and attack on social justice was happening in America, an identical event was occurring in Europe. In Germany the far-right party, AfD, achieved its best-ever result in the federal election held on 23rd February 2025, winning 20.8% of the vote and 152 seats to become the second-largest party. The AfD now joins with France's National Rally, Italy's Brothers of Italy, Poland's Law and Justice, Austria's Freedom Party, Hungary's Fidesz, and the UK's Reform UK in opposing progressive cultural policies across Europe.

As I explain in Chapter 3, there are many and varied reasons why people vote for particular parties, even when it may appear on the surface to be against their best interests to do so. A lot of women – and no doubt LGBTQ+ people too – will have voted for these right-wing, anti-feminist, anti-gay, anti-women politicians, though all the evidence suggests that it is young men, not young women, who are the key voting bloc behind this swing to the right.[2]

---

[1] https://www.wjbf.com/news/u-s-world-news/competent-white-men-must-be-in-charge-if-you-want-things-to-work-trump-admin-hires-darren-beattie-to-run-public-diplomacy-at-state-department/ https://www.theguardian.com/commentisfree/2025/feb/26/donald-trump-straight-white-men-diversity-kemi-badenoch-business-multiculturalism-economy

On which point, it would be interesting, if not highly disturbing, to see how much support Andrew Tate would receive should he ever decide to, or be eligible to, stand for election in the UK as he threatened to do at the time I was finishing this book.

While the likes of Trump, Musk and Tate are at least consistent and therefore predictable in their misogyny and anti-liberal position, one has to look elsewhere to see the deeper impact of male fundamentalism on society – for example your local McDonalds.

Companies scaling back or ending DEI initiatives, mostly since Donald Trump got re-elected in 2024, include:

- Meta (formerly Facebook)
- Walmart
- McDonalds
- Target
- PepsiCo
- Lowe's
- Harley-Davidson
- Boeing
- John Deere
- Uber
- Disney
- Paramount
- Molson Coors
- Brown-Foreman
- Accenture

One notable absentee from this list of corporate anti-DEI giants is Apple. In February 2025, CEO Tim Cook reaffirmed Apple's commitment to an inclusive workplace and DEI policies, and in doing so was overwhelmingly supported by Apple shareholders.

One likely outcome of the corporate backlash against feminism, diversity and, in essence, independent femininity, will be a rebranding, with terms such as 'inclusion', 'total inclusivity' and 'belonging' replacing DEI, the main reason being that companies fear DEI programmes negatively impacting their bottom line. And with some justification. There can be no doubt that young men constitute a massive global market and therefore, from a CEO's position, it makes no sense to alienate them. As Gillette discovered in

---

[2] https://www.bbc.com/news/articles/cy082dn7rkqo – Why more young men in Germany (and Europe) are turning to the far right.

January 2019, when it launched its highly controversial 'The Best Men Can Be' advertising campaign, aimed at addressing issues of toxic masculinity, bullying and sexual harassment, a lot of men don't want to be told they should hold each other accountable for their behaviour, not least when they are trimming their beards.

While these moves against women and LGBTQ+ people (and ethnic minorities) are worrying and must be resisted, in one way they are good. Because they serve to confirm and validate the arguments put forward by a legion of feminists, liberal thinkers, and gender theorists over the past seventy years, which is that there is abroad in the world a way of thinking about and living out manliness and masculinity which is damaging, oppressive, violent, and achieves its sense of purpose and existential validation from marginalising and oppressing 'others', notably women and LGBTQ+ people. Nothing Trump, Musk or Tate have done or said thus far would be of any surprise to the late Andrea Dworkin, Simone de Beauvoir or the currently very alive and active, Judith Butler.

The gender revolution has been around for a lot longer than any current politician; its signs and actors were visible long before the current tranche of 'strong men' were even born. And it will still be with us long after such individuals are gone. Women's desire for an independent, agentic, and safe life is not incumbent on any single individual, political party, government, or social trend. It is bigger than all that – and as I show in this book, it has history on its side. While there can be no doubt that a great many men, aided by some women, are a threat to the well-being, security, safety and aspirations of independent women, LGBTQ+ people and progressives everywhere, this is not a new condition: it is an ancient one. What is new is that gender has now become openly political – along with masculinity. This is just one consequence of the gender revolution and it is both welcome and irreversible. Every time the misogynist, homophobe, racist and hater expresses open contempt for 'others', they do the rest of us a great favour – by ditching their weasel words and finally revealing to the world just what they really believe and just who they really are.

None of which will do much to remove the wall now fast being erected between women and men. As I emphasise in this book, women and men are no longer living apart: they are growing apart. And the main reason is because women have changed and men have not. Sure, there are many men who have adapted willingly to the gender revolution and who have no problem rejecting toxic masculinity in all its many manifestations. Unfortunately, there are not enough such men to now save gender relations. Artificial Intelligence awaits and it will have its day.

Chapter 1: The Gender Revolution

I began writing this book on 18th October 2024, which happened to be the day the world awoke to the news that Hamas leader, Yahya Sinwar, had been killed by the Israeli Defence Force in Gaza.[3] On the face of it, this was not a news item one would directly connect to this book's themes, except for one aspect – the role that Israeli women will have directly or indirectly played in Sinwar's killing. You may not have heard of the IDF's Caracal Battalion unless you happen to be caught up in the Gaza/Israeli conflict, in which case you'll be well aware of the growing legend surrounding this lethal force, two-thirds of whom are women and which operates on the Gaza/Egyptian border, precisely where Sinwar was killed.[4]

During World War Two, the country with the highest percentage of women combat troops was Russia, though even they only constituted 1% of the Red Army. Over seven decades later and having women on the front line and fighting alongside men has become normalised; they are demonstrating their combat effectiveness and a deadly efficiency in a growing number of countries, not least Israel.[5]

For such a profound cultural shift to occur and over a relatively short time-span, two things need to happen: the first is individual women envisioning themselves killing their country's enemies; the second is a majority of men deciding they should be given the opportunity.

Note that the former must happen before the latter will respond. That is, women must first acquire an aspiration and vision together with the desire to turn that vision into reality. This then puts pressure on men to rethink their gendered behaviours and attitudes. History shows that men rarely if ever voluntarily open a door to women's ambitions – women always have to kick it open.

This reveals the power reality informing gender identities. Globally, men control the legal powers to kill, to decide who and when to kill, and to decide

---

[3] https://www.aljazeera.com/news/2024/10/18/hamas-confirms-leader-yahya-sinwar-killed-in-combat-in-gaza-by-israeli-army

[4] https://www.middleeastmonitor.com/20231213-report-israel-calls-up-female-battalion-for-special-tasks-in-gaza/

[5] https://en.wikipedia.org/wiki/Women_in_the_military_by_country

who will be permitted to do the killing. In other words, men dominate and control the armed forces, the police, the judiciary and the governments, together with all the attendant decision-making processes. Historically, a key aspect of men's entitlement and central therefore to constructions of traditional masculinity, has been their monopoly on the use of force.

However, no longer do men dominate these mechanisms of power 100%. They have had to relinquish power to women and are increasingly doing so. Women are kicking open doors with increasing force and increasing rapidity.[6]

This is just one indicator of an important fact very relevant to this book, which is that the gender revolution that has erupted over the past 75 years is one not driven by men but driven by women, albeit aided and abetted by a minority of men.

The transformation from women imagining themselves as housewives and mothers into – for example – lethal combat troops doesn't just upset the traditional gender power equation; it totally destroys the traditional gender identity equation of how men and women have over time come to think of themselves as gendered beings. This raises some interesting questions. For example, given that down the ages organised and random violence has not been a prevailing factor in the construction of femininity, how is it that large numbers of women around the world are now demanding the right to wear a uniform and tote a weapon? What 'gender abnormality' exists at the heart of this reformation of feminine identity?

The answer is that there is no abnormality – there is only the exercise of imagination and agency.

Firstly, the woman must be able to imagine herself as a trained professional killer and then have the agentic opportunity to create that as reality. In other words, the process is barely different to that which any similarly aspiring male soldier would go through.

Except for one important difference – men are over three times more likely than women to be perpetrators of violence. No cultural or existential chasm exists between soldiering and traditional masculinity; indeed, down through history, one has begat the other. This is in stark contrast to women, violence and femininity. For women to even begin to imagine themselves

---

[6] While weaponised AI creates risks for women, they are increasingly leveraging technology in defence roles. In the Ukraine, women lead in cybersecurity, AI-driven war crime documentation, and countering disinformation. https://www.stopkillerrobots.org/gender-and-killer-robots/

as combat troops they must first reimagine and then reinvent who they are as females – thereby creating a new type of femininity.

Take a pause and reflect on just what it means for a woman to recreate her femininity into a way of being, a sense of self that does not correspond with traditional gender values. Who will she model herself on? What narrative must she create for her emergent feminine identity? What social and political systems will provide her with support and validation? None of these questions is easily answered for any woman, though identifying what and who will resist her is not too difficult.

Any woman seeking to break free of the constraints of traditional femininity must first find the strength of will to overcome a great many resistances – not least familial, social, cultural, religious, political, economic and patriarchal. Arguably the biggest resistance will be located within herself, in her own sense of possibilities as a woman. Depending to what degree she has assimilated traditional femininity, so will her possibility for agency and action be determined.

The IDF's Caracal Battalion and women soldiers are not the focus of this book; they merely act as a timely illustration of the historic revolution in gender relations which has taken place over the past seven decades together with men's responses to it. Like every revolution down through history, the gender one has made waves. And being the biggest and most profound revolution ever in human history, the waves are – as you'd expect – now becoming quite large and powerful. Though as I suggest in this book, the biggest waves are yet to come and will certainly impact on us all. No matter who you are, where you live or what gender you present as, the gender revolution is making waves in your life and will make a good many more.

In examining the gender revolution, I am taking my main starting point as the 1950s, though that is not when it 'all began'. Truth is, no one knows when it all began. The gender revolution is not marked by an angry mob storming a Bastille or Winter Palace, nor by a political coup led by an ambitious colonel. It has been steadily emerging for centuries, though not in any uniform or linear way across every country and culture. Indeed, it may well be that this particular revolution has always been with us, has always had its principal actors and actresses, and has informed in a multitude of ways the best and worst of human experience down through history. But from the end of World War Two and certainly into the 1950s, something more radical and direct happened. Around the world, groups of women began to rise up and form an identifiable political entity with an equally identifiable political manifesto (feminism), thereby giving voice to their frustration and anger at the condition of gender relations, specifically what they termed 'patriarchy'. Some of the key moments, texts and actresses in the emergent feminist discourse of the 1950s and 1960s are examined in some detail in the following chapter, though this is not to suggest that women only found their voice in the 1950s. Women have always had a voice. They have always been able to exert some power – if not within a maleist[7] organisational system then at least in the private sphere. And they have never stopped dreaming, imagining and desiring.

But from the 1950s onwards, sparked by a number of aligning global, cultural, social and political conditions, one half of humanity (females) began to rapidly and forcefully reshape and recreate their sense of gender identity and in so doing directly challenged the power and gender identity of the other half of humanity – the males.

We are now 75 years into the dynamics of this revolution: this may sound a lot, but in terms of humanity's presence on earth (now around 200,000 years) is but a tiny fraction. Indeed, it is the span of a single lifetime, mine for example. The gender revolution may have been a long time coming and for millennia its signs gone largely unnoticed by the masses and their leaders, but in the past 75 years all that quietness, invisibility and accompanying complacency, at least on the part of men, has been swept aside. There is now, not surprisingly, a lot of noise around gender: and for many men, fear.[8] This is hardly surprising because as far as men and their masculinities are concerned, over the past two decades the historic silence surrounding that particular personal/social arrangement has been totally blown away.

We do indeed live through interesting and historic times when 'all that once appeared stable and solid melts into air', and what is certainly melting into air is the traditional gender identity binary along with the powers, assumptions, and values which have hitherto enabled it.

Differences and Compulsions

Having just declared the demise of the gender binary I am now compelled to acknowledge the reality, which is that we all continue to perpetuate it, not least myself in the writing of this book. Men and women, female and male, femininities and masculinities are unavoidable social anchors. Not only do they help us categorise this diverse world, they provide potent and

---

[7] Maleist: Biased towards males, dominated by males, conforms to a traditional masculine culture.

[8] See for examples and discussion, Butler, J. (2024) Who's Afraid of Gender", London: Penguin.

persuasive political standpoints and it is upon these gender standpoints that I ground this book. Therefore, in declaring that 'women rose up' from the 1950s onwards, one shouldn't take that as a global absolute. Not all women stormed the barricades of male privilege, nor are they doing so today. Likewise, when I detail the male responses to the gender revolution in Chapter 4, it will be clear that not all men are resisting: many are active supporters, not least myself as long-time pro-feminist man.

Just like any revolution, the gender one draws its supporters, advocates and detractors from across the social spectrum; individuals whom one would not expect to be seen crossing particular political gender lines continue to do so. This should not altogether surprise us once we recognise that there are as many differences within the categories of male and female as there are between the categories of male and female. If there is one sure thing in this world, it is that no two humans are exactly alike. Whatever our personal, political and social preferences and gravitations, we each remain unique from our neighbour.

That said, the politics of gender identity does not permit such an easy escape for the individual; we are only allowed so much fluidity. Even as a growing number of governments loosen up on their gender binary requirement for the official identification of their citizens, i.e. for issuing passports and ID cards, we still have to contend with the social conventions and those conventions for the most part remain comfortable with the idea of men and women, male and female, along with many of the corresponding stereotypes and assumptions which serve to reify these dualities.

Indeed, even those individuals self-declared as LGBTQ+ tend (though not in every case) to demand legal and social association with the half of the gender binary to which they feel they belong, a conundrum currently being played out with increasing vocal ferocity in liberal societies especially: i.e. what is a 'woman'? Who should be allowed and under what conditions to be identified as such, and who should not?[9] In a very real way, the gender revolution has flung open the door to such discussions and contestations, thereby contributing to the 'queering' of society[10] not least by spotlighting emergent and pre-existing differences within humanity, giving voice

---

[9] For discussion on free speech in universities and, relatedly, whether 'Trans Women are Women' see Whitehead, S. and O'Connor, P. (2022) *Creating a Totally Inclusive University*. London: Routledge. Chapter 10.

[10] I'm using the term 'queering' in the poststructuralist understanding of it. See, for examples, Corber, R. J. and Valocchi, S. (eds) (2003) *Queer Studies: An Interdisciplinary Reader*. Oxford: Blackwell Publishing.

and energy to those differences together with a vibrant political (usually feminist) platform from which to fight for equality, inclusion, justice – and visibility.

This passionate desire of humans to associate and connect tells us that while it is correct to recognise the reality of over eight billion unique individuals, it is unwise to assume all eight billion want to be isolated in their uniqueness. If we humans have one innate compulsion it is to belong and gender provides us with a very powerful belonging possibility. To be labelled male or female at birth can be a major problem for some – notably the intersex and those who identify as transgender and non-binary – but for the rest it is the basis around which they will willingly build their life. The vast majority of humans identified at birth as female or male have absolutely no desire or intention to change that fact.

This book is, therefore, concerned with women and men as two distinct political/social gender categories rather than as biological fixtures and examines the future of these two categories based on a revolution initiated by one of them: the female/woman. Women may remain the 'second sex' in many parts of the world, but as far as the gender revolution is concerned, they own it and they are driving it. However, this revolution is not only of concern to the two dominant sexes nor is it only challenging the two most traditional expressions of gender identity: hegemonic masculinity and hegemonic femininity. Every other possible gender and sex compilation is implicated also. As stated above, the gender revolution excludes no one and no one can avoid its impact, which tells us that while this revolution is very similar to every other revolution created by humanity – notably in its quest for a fair and just division of resources, powers and spaces together with an end to oppression, discrimination and violence – at its heart is something much less tangible: identity.

The Sociology of Identity

This book is not offered as a sociological text nor written primarily for those in academia, though hopefully (some of) the academy will read it. Nevertheless, given that I am examining gender and identity, along with the powers which circulate within and around feminine and masculine performances, it would be erroneous to omit any reference to theory: identity doesn't just emerge on the wind – it has origins and these origins need to be illuminated.

The theoretical basis to this book, indeed to all my work on gender, is feminist poststructuralism, which I summarise as follows:

> 'Feminist post-structuralism emphasises the multiple, contingent and fluid aspects of the self and our sense of identity... stressing that gender is not a biological or predicted outcome but a process configured by the repetition of performative [discursive] acts undertaken by the individual, albeit not necessarily with cognisance of these acts.'[11]

Everything which follows in these pages is informed directly or indirectly by the above theory and understanding of how individuals acquire an identity, become a gender and learn to express their unique gendered self. It would not serve the aims of this book to delve any deeper into feminist poststructuralism as there are far better texts available for that purpose.[12] But it is important to establish the theoretical basis on which I proceed to examine gender, identity, women and men and all associated concepts.

One of the most influential conceptual offspring of feminist poststructuralism is intersectionality.[13] This is a more recent feminist theory which I explain as follows:

> '[Intersectionality]... recognises that each individual identity exists at the intersections of many aspects of self and social powers; encourages the recognition that gender intersects with (for example) race, sex, sexuality, ability, ethnicity, age, culture and class to 'produce' the individual; and that, as discrete forms of oppression, these variables combine to have a powerful impact on women's lives in ways which may not always be apparent to the individual.'[14]

To summarise the above: every individual now and who has ever lived has an identity constituted by multiple social variables including gender, age, class and race. These intersect to produce the individual but not in any absolute, predictable or biologically determined fashion. The individual is a discursive subject, created through language and action, narrative

---

[11] Whitehead, S., Talahite, A. and Moodley, R. (2013) *Gender and Identity*. Oxford: Oxford University Press. p. 90

[12] See for examples see; Weedon, C. (2003) *Feminist Practice and Poststructuralist Theory*. London: Blackwell. Sarup, M. (1993) *An Introductory Guide to Post-Structuralism and Postmodernism*. London: Harvester Wheatsheaf.

[13] See, Collins, P.H. and Bilge, S. (2020) *Intersectionality*. Cambridge: Polity.

[14] Whitehead, S et al, (2013). p. 91

and embodiment, culture and symbolism. The individual is in flux, has a fluid and alterable identity, and is forever in a dynamic state of being and becoming.

In short, we are all culturally informed, contingent and inhabiting multiple identity variables. This explains why it can be a challenge to feel grounded and fixed either within our selves or in our respective society.

This is where femininity and masculinity come in.

The Sociology of Masculinity and Femininity

From the moment of our birth and pronouncement of our sex identity, an unquantifiable array of gendered discourses proceeds to envelop us. These languages, behaviours, stories, narratives, actions, assumptions, symbols and signs provide the child with what sociologists term a 'discursive subject position'. This may sound complicated but basically it means we humans plant each innocent newly born child in a particular gendered pot, labelled male or female, and proceed to water and feed it with gendered discourses (language, actions, stereotypes, expectations), a bit like a houseplant. The child duly grows within that pot and in the process assimilates the ways being expected of her or him.

Sure, there are a growing number of parents who are only too well aware of this process and who try to avoid it, but doing so isn't easy. Parents do have a massive and profound influence on their offspring but so too does social media, smartphones, videos and schoolmates.

And then there is the sexuality element, recognised by most sociologists as having a biological basis and therefore of limited fluidity; we are born straight, gay or bi and not much – if anything – will change that fact.

One can now recognise how we arrive at the unique complexity of individuality, it being due to all these intersecting components feeding information into our consciousness and subconsciousness like a permanently active transport system, some of which is biologically based but most of which is social influence. Every person on earth spends their life living out this complexity and trying to make sense of it.

If you have been wondering where the gender binary fits into all this, then here is your answer:

By being identified as male or female, so does the growing child assimilate the discourses associated with the gender binary, with the 'discursive subject

---

[15] For definition and explanation of these terms see, Whitehead, S.M. (2001) *Men and Masculinities.* Cambridge, Polity. Chapter 7

position' mentioned above separating into either a 'masculine subject position' or a feminine subject position'.[15]

Basically, both masculinity and femininity can be defined as follows:

> 'Masculinities and femininities are those actions, languages and practices existing in specific cultural and organisational locations, which are commonly associated with how masculine males and feminine females are expected to behave. By being thus culturally defined, the behaviour of men and women is designed, and expected to be, differentiated.'[16]

As I detail throughout the book, but especially in Chapters 3 and 4, masculinities and femininities both play a major role in the direction and consequences of the gender revolution, not least because it is through these gendered, and thereby politicised, discursive subject positions that the individual achieves some sense of being and belonging.

There can be crossover between these gendered subject positions and – as we know from LGBTQ+ identities – a large number of individuals don't fit neatly into any social/sexual box, but in the final reckoning most of the eight billion people on earth are slotted into this gender binary, willing or not.

The takeaway from this brief examination of gender identity is that both masculinity and femininity are multiple, fluid constructs or influences; there is more than one masculinity and more than one femininity but all such performances are a product of social and cultural dynamics or, in sociological terms, discourses. However, as I discuss in the following chapters, there are some ways of being a man which have assumed dominance over time, and likewise ways of being a woman. These dominant masculinities and dominant femininities have not come about nor been created by chance but by force, persuasion, design, rhetoric and, most important, by the exercise of power.

Understanding Power

An everyday understanding of power envisages it operating as a hierarchy, with the most 'powerful' at the top and below them progressively declining levels of individual power leading to those of us at the very bottom of the social heap. While this is instantly recognisable, it is a flawed and limited understanding of how power works. We all have power to some degree.

---

[16] Adapted from Whitehead, S.M. and Barrett, F.J. (eds) (2001) *The Masculinities Reader.* Cambridge: Polity. (Introduction)

Creating our individuality, our particular identity mix, requires power and agency. And even the so-called 'powerful' cannot assume it – there are myriad ways in which power can be lost as well as gained. We cannot bank and accumulate power like we do money. Nor can we pass it down to our children like property and gold. Power circulates; it is discursive, linguistic, knowledge-related, and affected by how we present ourselves to others. This is especially so in today's hyper-sensitive globalised media world when the famous and the powerful can be pulled down very quickly, say by simply posting an inappropriate message on Facebook, Instagram, Tik Tok or X.[17]

This is why I have elsewhere written critically about the idea of gender power and patriarchy being rigid, fixed and unchallengeable.

> *'...despite the potency of such concepts [i.e. patriarchy, gender order and hegemonic masculinity] and the emotiveness they engender, they have fundamental inconsistencies and weaknesses for understanding the dynamic and fluid relationships between political categories of gender and between individual women and men. Most notable in this regard is their inability to provide a theory of the (gendered) subject (individual) as an active yet constrained factor in the reproduction of dominance, and in the resistance to dominance.'*[18]

Today, there are countless examples of women exerting power and agency both in their public and private lives and some of these I examine in depth in Chapter 5. Indeed, women's ability to exert power is fundamental to the gender revolution. All of which undermines male assumptions of superiority as well as any misunderstandings men may have about their biological primacy over women. It is worth reflecting on how global society has managed to find itself in the midst of a gender revolution led by women, when many men and some women consider male power to be an absolute, totalising (if not biologically inevitable) and natural state. In short, according to the beliefs of a lot of traditional men, the gender revolution is a biological impossibility. As with all revolutions, the gender one has taken people by surprise, not least those men who thought their male privilege, or what has been termed a 'patriarchal dividend',[19] could never be challenged or reduced.

---

[17] Examples at time of writing: https://www.buzzfeed.com/aronawriting/celebrity-stupid-social-media-posts-downfall https://www.watchmojo.com/articles/top-20-celebs-who-destroyed-their-careers-with-one-post

[18] Whitehead, S.M. (2001) p.p.110-111

This book is not the place to closely examine the intricacies and contradictions inherent in power, but it is important to note that without power women cannot change anything in their lives. Very obviously they are changing a lot of things, not least themselves, and to do that they need power or, as I also term it in this book, agency.

Another interesting aspect of power is that it is rarely if ever equally distributed; it moves, flows, and has its very own complex gravitational pull. I have long recognised that for women to gain power (agency) men would have to lose it; as far as the gender revolution is concerned, this *is* a zero-sum game.

Why? Because the power that men have felt in their lives – indeed traditional masculinity itself – is based on having power over women; especially authority and control of resources, organisations, wealth, government, law and violence with women marginalised in respect of all these elements. Once women rise up and take some of that power, occupy powerful positions and exert influence over society and assume authority for themselves, then inevitably men will have to lose out. Imagine it like a pair of scales with women taking from the men's side of the power scale and depositing power on their own side. Will there ever be an equalising? I doubt it – this is one set of scales which will keep moving up and down.

That said, throughout this book I use terms which indicate male power; notably, patriarchy, hegemonic masculinity, gender order, maleism, and masculinism.[20] This is a literary device enabling me to distinguish how power impacts the two main gender political categories – it is not meant to be deterministic nor to suggest that any of these male power mechanisms are natural and inviolate.

A final point about power is how it relates to individual subjectivity. It is very revealing that research into children's expression of self invariably shows that boys – even at kindergarten – imagine themselves to be smarter, stronger and superior to girls.[21] This subjective differentiation from the opposite sex does not arise from biology: in terms of physical strength,

---

[19] How the patriarchal system serves men's interests directly or indirectly. See R.W. Connell (2003) *Masculinities*. Cambridge: Polity.

[20] Masculinism: From the work of Arthur Brittan, and meaning 'the ideology that justifies and naturalises male domination… the ideology of patriarchy'. Brittan, A. (1989) *Masculinity and Power*. Oxford: Basil Blackwell.

[21] https://www.forbes.com/sites/gaudianohunt/2017/01/30/even-six-year-olds-know-it-working-hard-is-better-than-being-smart/   https://www.sydney.edu.au/

there is no difference between male and female until puberty and as far as 'cleverness' is concerned, females now outperform males across the educational spectrum from kindergarten to PhD,[22] Instead, it comes from the male's desire to be better and believing themselves so, despite all the evidence to the contrary.

Such a desire is a very tentative, if not risky, base on which to build gender identity and a secure sense of (masculine) self. The gender revolution is now disclaiming and destroying these gendered assumptions, not just for children but for adult men especially. This leaves men without the power they imagined, believed in, and indeed were taught they were entitled to. For those men unable to adjust to the new gender reality, retreat into male fundamentalism is almost inevitable, though as I explain in Chapter 4, such a move would be a sad indictment of men's weaknesses.

That said, the gender revolution is not divesting men of all their power: while they are losing some material power and their power over women, they will still have the power to reflect, self-analyse, consider, and adjust their masculinity so as to compliment, not conflict with, women's new-found aspirations and expressions of femininity. Of course, that will take courage and self-confidence. It will also take self-awareness and an ability to recognise and then disassociate from the multitude of myths, falsehoods, delusions and fallacies which have long embedded themselves in traditional notions of gender identity. The whole idea of gender political categories – 'natural differences between men and women' – draws on a host of such myths and misconceptions. Some of these are actively promoted by men who intend to retain power and authority over women (e.g. misogynists); some are actively promoted by those who have political agendas, notably right-wing propagandists; and some people, women and men, actively promote them because their whole identity and sense of self is invested in discourses and ideologies (e.g. religions) that, whether they realise it or not, serve to position men over women.

---

news-opinion/news/2017/08/04/when-it-comes-to-sport--boys-play-like-a-girl.html https://thinkorblue.com/gender-stereotypes-in-schools/

[22] https://www.forbes.com/sites/nickmorrison/2024/01/14/from-kindergarten-to-college-girls-are-outperforming-boys/ https://www.applerouth.com/blog/troubling-gender-gaps-in-education https://spartanshield.org/42176/feature/its-a-girls-world/

Chapter 1: The Gender Revolution

Agency not Biology

One of the realisations brought forth by the gender revolution and its supporters, especially gender theorists, is that biology is not destiny. Sex, sexuality and gender do not determine our possibilities, our potential, even while they influence our life and our sense of identity. We each have agency, though to grasp that self-power and make it work for us means first letting go of many 'comforting' delusions. This is especially true for women who love men, who desire men, who believe they need men in their life, and who have hitherto been prepared to sacrifice their own opportunities and circumscribe their own lives in order to keep men happy. One of the arguments put forward in this book is that the gender revolution, and the desire for independent femininity which is elementary to it, challenges if not changes heterosexual women's relationship to men and their need for them. Some may consider this 'sad', others may consider it 'hopeful', but either way, this is one of the inevitable consequences of women as a gender group exercising agency, power and choice for the first time in history. Women around the world are now actively creating a new gender narrative, one which does not have men at its centre.

In the final analysis, and for reasons I explain in the book, no one can escape the consequences of the gender revolution, even if they hope to. This is one revolution that is not going to dissolve into the social atmosphere; end up being corrupted by some maniacal colonel, a Stalin or a Hitler; or be forgotten by all but future historians. And yet its very magnitude and import serve to confuse and disturb: how to make sense of something so massive, so global, so personal and so far-reaching? How to lock onto the global picture when it is mighty difficult to see even the local one? One way is to simply recognise and accept that for millennia, the gender binary, traditional sex roles, and the unchallenged dominance of men served to configure and construct society. That is now finishing, coming to an end. Today we are fast heading into a world where all that which gave us a (patriarchal) structure and a (patriarchal) purpose are no more. None of which confirms where we are now heading. I've spent half my life, over 35 years, examining this structure from a sociological perspective and even I cannot be sure what happens next. But there are indicators and these are examined. I think we can all agree on what has happened because the evidence tells us, and a great many of us will agree on why it has happened, though that will possibly depend on which side of the binary we sit. But as to where we are heading, whether to the End of Sex or some other place, you'll decide for yourself.

Have I written this book for you?

Although I am a declared feminist, or pro-feminist male, I have not written this book only for feminists, who I describe as follows:

> *'If you believe in equality for women, are pro LGBTQ+, consider that all societies must challenge male abuse, and de facto, educate males into less violent and damaging forms of behaviour, then you are a feminist. Therefore, to not be a feminist is to not seek a change in men's behaviour nor seek the advancement of women to a state of independence from men.'*[23]

Whether you are one of the many millions of women (and men) who align with feminism or not, if you are even remotely concerned at the current state of gender relations then you should hopefully get some benefit from reading my analysis and conclusions regarding the global gender revolution. And after reading, perhaps you'll realise you are a lot more of a feminist than you previously imagined.

Neither, as a Western boomer, am I writing only for Westerners drawing – or about to draw – their pension. I am presenting a global analysis and while it could be argued that the gender revolution has been nourished by the growth of Western feminism, there can be no doubt that it is impacting every corner on earth. Indeed, as I discuss, some regions – East Asia and India in particular – may even now be leading it, especially Gen Z Asian women.

In terms of my own slow awakening to feminism both as theory and practice, that began when I was aged forty and engaged in a part-time MA in sociology in Leeds, UK. Back then, I was already a full-time educator (Lecturer in a Further Education College) and acquiring a heightened understanding of race and class dynamics, but even so, feminism was certainly a step beyond my comfort zone. Once I overcame my wariness about feminism and feminists, and started to shake off forty years of acquired myths and stereotypes regarding the 'naturalness' of women and men, there was no stopping me. This will be my twentieth book so perhaps for me, "writin' is indeed fightin'".[24] Certainly, there have been times when

---

[23] Original definition in Whitehead, S. (2021) *Toxic Masculinity: Curing the Virus.* London: AG Books.

[24] The phrase "Writin' is Fightin'" is attributed to Ishmael Reed, an American poet, novelist, essayist and activist. Reed used this phrase as titlte of his 1988 collection

my urge to write felt like that. But not with this book. This book is written not only as a contribution to the gender revolution but as a wake-up call for all of us. Although I am a full supporter of the gender revolution and have been for several decades, I don't see all good coming from its outcomes. I cannot claim to be enthused by the prospect of AI relationships and the displacement of human intimacy with that of human/machine intimacy, as explored in Chapter 6. Nor am I persuaded that much good will arise from seeing some countries and cultures disappear due to severely declining birth rates. At the same time, this revolution looks and feels inevitable, and for the most part I certainly welcome it, though as with every revolution that humans have instigated, the outcomes may not entirely match the hopes.

Just as I have done, every individual reader will decide where they stand in relation to this historic shift in gender power and reformation of gender and sexual relationships. Perhaps reading this book will not change many people's views; if they are liberal regarding gender relationships, perhaps even feminist, then they'll remain so. If they are male fundamentalists then my book won't make for a reassuring read, in which case they may well retreat further into their opposition to women and their independent feminine identity.

And what about the reader sitting on the fence; the individual unsure as to whether they are for or against a new independent femininity and all it will usher in? Well, my question to you is 'do you want to be on the right side of history or not?', because there is no going back to the past as far as gender relationships are concerned. Far better to embrace the future and try to steer it in the least violent and non-toxic direction. In short, I hope what follows – my arguments and evidence – will provide you with a better understanding and appreciation of the most far-reaching and profound revolution ever to impact human society, and spur you to contribute positively to ensuring it brings the best, not worse, for all of us. Because the dramatic social changes that I detail in this book are already with us and impacting around the world. There is no avoiding them, there is only understanding them and then working out the most effective way of handling them, maximising their positive potential while reducing their negative impact on us all.

---

of essays, etc, covering 37 years of his writing career. https://www.goodreads.com/en/book/show/985349.Writin_Is_Fightin_?t

How the book is Organised, Written and Structured

Having read this far, you will have realised that for me the gender revolution is more than a sociological phenomenon to be dryly analysed. It is very much a personal, lived story; vivid, colourful, emotive and highly impactful. This book, then, is not about regurgitating and presenting evidence but about telling a story. This is why I have written it as a personal/political/intellectual narrative, interweaving snippets of sociological theory and scholarly literature with the social (media, popular culture, narratives, anecdotes) and the personal – my autobiography. The personal – my reflections – is especially apparent in Chapter 2, where I look at the rise of feminism between 1950 and 1990, charting my own formative journey through these decades, while noting my distance from that which would eventually come to define my later life. The 1950s are significant not just because this decade saw the tentative early globalisation of feminist enquiry, but also because it was my first decade. Until I began writing this book I hadn't fully appreciated that Simone de Beauvoir published *The Second Sex* in 1949, the year of my birth.[25] A nice coincidence and one which encouraged me to frame my story with the emergent gender revolution.

As Chapter 3 reveals, my distance from feminism and feminists disappeared very quickly once the 90s got underway. This period of personal awakening coincided, at least as I came to understand it, with the rise of independent femininity as a global narrative for empowered, agentic, self-actualising womanhood. The term 'independent femininity' as I define it is mine, though in truth it belongs to every woman. I have simply put a name to that which women around the world are creating for themselves. For the purposes of this book and my argument, I needed to define what my research and experiences were telling me – which is that feminism as a global discourse was displaced, certainly from the 1990s onwards, by a way of being a woman which was feminist at its core but without the ideological implications and political labelling. I struggled to come up with a 'creative' term to describe this new, modern femininity – 'unfettered', 'agentic', 'positive', 'liberated' and 'enlightened' were some options – though in the end I stuck with 'independent' because this really describes it so neatly. But independent from what, exactly? Well, two things, both identities themselves; traditional femininity and its symbiotic 'twin',

---

[25] de Beauvoir, S. (1953) [1949] *The Second Sex*. New York: Vintage. The book was originally banned by the Vatican.

traditional masculinity. The former is defined and detailed in Chapter 3, the latter is examined in Chapter 4.

The Oxford English Dictionary defines 'revolution' as '*a period or instance of significant change or radical alteration of a particular condition, state of affairs'… the complete overthrow of an established government or social order by those previously subject to it.*'

Based on this definition, it is self-evident that global society is in the throes of a gender revolution, has been for some decades and may well be for some time to come. Will we ever get to the 'complete overthrow' of the patriarchal social order around the world? I don't know and nor does anyone else, but the direction is unmistakeable. This leaves many questions, one of which concerns how men are responding to the rise of women, the growing ubiquity of independent femininity, and the revolution itself. In Chapter 4, I examine 'men's responses' from the 1970s to the present day. Many years ago, I was writing and researching on how men were responding to feminism and identified the key responses as 'for', 'against', 'hiding' and 'confused'. These four responses hold true to this day, though in this chapter I am primarily concerned with three types of men; the male fundamentalists, the traditionalists, and the progressives.

I first noted that women and men were not only 'living apart but growing apart' in my 2021 book *Toxic Masculinity*, and some of the data and arguments presented in that book have turned out to be a rehearsal for a much fuller and detailed examination of what is nowadays recognised to be – and described by many commentators and researchers as – a 'global gender divergence'. Chapter 5 takes a very close look at this divergence in all its many forms: singletons, single motherhood, childlessness, marriage, birth rates, divorce, cohabitation, celibacy, bisexuality, mistrust and intimate partner violence, politics, and physical space. At the conclusion to this chapter, which incidentally is also framed around my family's history, I state what for me is the obvious result of the gender revolution – women and men going their separate ways. For a great number of individuals, that separation has been underway for some time and become permanent.

So where does that leave women and men? With regards to humanity's journey, there is no data available on what happens tomorrow or next year, and the end of the century is a complete mystery to all of us. We have to experience it first. But we can speculate. Chapter 6 is my speculation, albeit informed by what is now occurring around the world, but especially in the West and in East Asia, with regards to Artificial Intelligent 'partners'. I cannot claim to be optimistic about where the merging of the AI revolution with the gender revolution takes human society, but then neither am I wholly pessimistic. What I am is wary and cautious. In this chapter I provide evidence for both perspectives. What I do see looming up very fast is the end of sex as humans have traditionally understood it and experienced it. When humanity looks back on this era and recognises how the end of sex came about, it will be able to see the dual impact of gender divergence and AI technology.

Regarding terminology, although I use the terms 'women' and 'men' throughout the book, I am primarily concerned with cisgender (heterosexual) women and cisgender (heterosexual) men: individuals whose internal sense of gender corresponds with the sex they were identified as having at birth and whose main sexual attraction is to the opposite sex, though as I note in Chapter 5, it may be that cisgender straight women are a lot more sexually fluid than has ever been assumed. I am, therefore, not *primarily* examining the impact of the gender revolution on lesbian, gay, bisexual, transgender, and/or gender expansive, queer and/or questioning, intersex, asexual and two-spirit, nor LGBTQIA2S+ members' contribution to it. Such an examination deserves a thorough discussion and another book, though not one I feel qualified to write. This distinction is not made because of the lack of importance of these communities, but simply in order to retain throughout this book the dominant narrative of the gender political binary and (global) contestation between (cis)women and (cis) men, with their heterosexuality recognised as a powerful variable in the gender revolution.

I have deliberately limited the theoretical component in the book, and where unavoidable used it in simplified ways and/or via footnotes, though perhaps not always successfully. As one reader of draft chapters put it; 'even your explanation and definition of 'hegemonic' is a bit of a 'snake pit'![26] In my defence and as a long-time sociologist, it is impossible for me to write a book such as this without drawing on words and terms common to my intellectual field, such as 'discourse', 'hegemonic', and 'gendered subject'. Footnotes have hopefully aided interpretation for the reader without a sociological background, which will definitely be most.

Similarly, and as I observe in Chapter 5, the sheer volume of hard data supporting the many aspects of the gender revolution, independent femininity, men's responses, and especially the global gender divergence, is becoming overwhelming. It would not help create a readable narrative if even a fraction of these data were included in the book. Nevertheless, some

---

[26] I took Dr Cropper's advice and change my definition of hegemony to a more simplified version.

data, as supporting evidence, must be included and is. Wherever possible and wherever my writing skills allow, the data are included but without detriment, I hope, to the larger story – which is that women have changed. Now it is men's turn.

Chapter 2: Reflections on the Rise of Feminism: 1950 to 1990

In this chapter I take a very personal look at the rise of feminism and feminist theory since 1949 – the year of my birth – while also drawing on key evidence and events to show how the gender revolution progressed in the USA and UK during the four decades to 1990. As the chapter reveals, in many respects I am a child of feminism and certainly of independent femininity – something I have only recently come to appreciate – while also being influenced by the sexual revolution of the 1960s and 80s Thatcherism. My journey is mine alone, but much of it is not unique. To some extent, we are now all children of feminism and certainly of the gender revolution.

Born to be Feminist?
I was raised by feminists: I just didn't realise it at the time. But then nor did the women who raised me. They were strong personalities, independent-minded, not cowering under the patriarchal yoke and quite capable of voicing their opinions. One was a wealthy, rather imposing, Edwardian middle-class spinster who much later I came to recognise was a closet lesbian. Another was an aunt who, from the 1950s, built a highly successful business and eventually retired to the Isle of Man, a tax-exiled multimillionaire. She also managed to raise four children. Then there was my mother who, at age fourteen, was a full-time maid for a doctor and his family in 1930s Blackburn, Lancashire and whose last job, in her seventies, was cleaning the home of an opera singer in Southport, Merseyside. Between these eras she raised three children and managed a business with my father. I had a Nan, not a relative, who was devoted to me and became a close friend until she passed away when I was fifteen. One of her biggest thrills in life was buying a fur coat when her late husband's life insurance paid out. Finally, there was a fourth aunt who married a "rather dodgy" French-Canadian after WWII, went to live with him in the frozen north of Canada in the 1950s and died an alcoholic in a US trailer-park, aged 62. She was a woman who pushed at the boundaries. My family called her 'free-spirited' and 'fun-loving', which I came to learn was code for dangerous and unreliable. In the early 1950s she'd

walk around the genteel Edwardian coastal resort of Southport in trousers. Local women used to gossip about that – disapproval mixed with envy – though to be fair my aunt was pushing the limits; until the late 1960s the 'grandest restaurants in New York and Washington banned women from wearing trousers'.[27] The generation of women who bore and raised these 'feminists' – my grandmothers – were equally if not more tough, resilient and full of fortitude. They had to be.

You'll note that I left the men out of the picture. The truth is, there's not much to say about them: grandfathers, uncles, and my father. They were omnipresent but a tad irrelevant; the hard graft was done by the women. By the time I was ten (1960) I'd realised which gender was the strongest, the most caring and the most reliable; it wasn't the males.

But it wasn't entirely the fault of the men – they were beaten down by their traditional masculinity and the unrealistic expectations it placed upon them. They too were victims of the prevailing gender order:

> "I have loved men who were trapped by these expectations. Men who wanted to be tender but didn't know how to, who carried pain they couldn't even name, and who didn't have the words to speak it out loud. I've seen how silence and suppression erode their emotional wellbeing."[28]

My two grandfathers fought in WWI; virile young men eager to respond to Kitchener's call-up. Both survived physically but not mentally or emotionally. One died at 41, an alcoholic. The other took himself off from his growing family for long periods, leaving my grandmother to raise their three daughters alone. But beaten down or not, none of the adult men in my life was ever prepared to admit it. I suspect they cried silent tears in the dark, each having to deal with his own particular misery. They'd been raised to be masters and that is how they saw themselves; 'masters' of their home – the patriarch. They self-elevated to a position of dominance over the much more capable and durable women in their lives. Traditional masculinity worked its magic on these men, transforming them from losers to winners, at least in their imagination. In reality, they were not masters of very much at all, especially not themselves, and they knew it. As the years went by and these male relatives aged, I noticed how they grew quieter, more docile

---

[27]   Purnell, S. (2024) *Kingmaker: Pamela Churchill Harriman's astonishing life of seduction, intrigue and power.* London: Virago. P. 271.

[28]   Graham, M. (2024) *Modern Men.* Unpublished article sent to author, October.

and more vulnerable. The women, by contrast, aged differently; they grew stronger, more vocal, more confident – and happier.

One big difference between women and men in the 1950s was self-awareness, self-knowledge and self-understanding. The women had it; the men lacked it. It was as if the men went through life only partly awake, hiding behind a stoic, muscular Christianity[29] which left them emotionally inadequate but needing to appear strong. Whatever model of manliness they were striving for, they never quite achieved it. These men lived with a sense of incompleteness. Maybe it was grief. Today we'd call it PTSD. Like most young men who survived the world wars, my male relatives had had enough of military masculinity.[30] They were members of a brutalised generation of men who now yearned for release from drills, orders, death, destruction and trauma. From Britain to Germany, the USA to India, Japan to Italy, millions of men willingly went home from the battlefields in 1945 and ditched their uniforms. Whether on the winning or losing side, they now had to survive and they had to thrive. Corporate cigar-smoking masculinity or bureaucratic bowler-hatted masculinity awaited the lucky ones; the rest – stuck with a truculent working-class manliness – somehow had to muddle through in what was a rapidly changing world. But for a short period at least, they could imagine themselves as heroes.

For a great many men, 1945 didn't see the end of it: China, Korea, Vietnam, Egypt, Pakistan/India, Israel/Palestine, Indonesia and Malaysia were just some of the barely known places where conflict and war continued to draw men in, along with increasing numbers of women.

I and others of my generation, post-war boomers, can look back on the 1950s with some nostalgia, or at least we can if we're Brits. We were a lucky generation, born in peacetime and blessed to live mostly safe and healthy lives. Once we'd got through food rationing and the first televisions arrived, our world coloured up.[31] I cannot say the same for the rest of the

---

[29] 'Muscular Christian' manliness in the Victorian and Edwardian eras, defined as 'openly 'not feminine', more directly associated with physical strength, muscularity, physical trial, denial (of luxury) and 'endurance in the face of death and torment.' Whitehead, 2001, p, 14. From Newsome, D. (1961) *Godliness and Good Learning*. London: Routledge.

[30] Morgan, D.H.L. (2006) Theater of war: Combat, the military, and masculinities. In S.Whitehead (ed) *Men and Masculinities: Critical concepts in sociology*. (Vol.2). London: Routledge.

[31] Rationing finally ended in the UK in 1954. My parents bought their first television in 1956.

world as it desperately tried to emerge from the ashes not just of WWII but of disintegrating European colonies, civil wars and indigenous people's growing cry for freedom, typically in places were white men had ruled for centuries.

But as ever, it was men doing the fighting, causing the conflict and crying for freedom. The women were mostly silent or silenced. There was no global feminist movement in the early 1950s and therefore there were no feminists – at least declared as such. As in my family, many women had a feminist subjectivity; they just didn't have a language for it and couldn't name it. And by not being able to name it, they couldn't identify with it.

It would have been a thankless task to talk to most women in the 1950s about female empowerment, patriarchal conditions or equality of opportunity. After all, the two genders got along OK. They were falling in love, getting married, having children, and divorce was a rare experience. Populations were growing in most every country, fuelled by rising prosperity and a post-war urge to replenish humanity with a new generation untarnished by war and conflict.

On the surface, men and women were fulfilling their 'God-given roles', a functional arrangement that to many male sociologists of the day seemed entirely inevitable and natural.[32] Family life was the bedrock of society, it seemed, and the perfect family was nuclear with dad as breadwinner. The two genders were not in conflict – they were self-supporting, complementary and blessed with an inevitable heterosexuality.

This only goes to show how easily people are fooled into cooperating with the very ideologies which oppress them.

The men were living the myth and falsehood of male hegemony. The women were living the myth and falsehood of grateful domesticity.

Neither sex discussed any of this amongst themselves nor with their partners – gender, sex and sexuality did not make for polite conversation in the 1950s, though under this domestic tranquillity there were rumblings.

The 51% Minority Other

At exactly the time I was beginning my traditional, highly didactic northern English primary school education, an American sociologist,

---

[32] For example, Talcot Parsons and his theory of structural functionalism; a sociological perspective that views society as a set of coherent parts that work together to create social order and equilibrium. Parson. C. (1951) *The Social System*. New York: The Free Press.

Helen Mayer Hacker, was making history. In 1951 she had published *Women as a Minority Group*[33] and in so doing began the dismantling of the myths around traditional sex and gender roles. Her research into women's marginalisation and her liberal feminist analysis as to how patriarchy positioned women at the edges of society, made a major contribution to first-wave feminist theory, eventually opening the door to women's studies in Western universities.

Before the 1950s were over, Hacker was to make an arguably even bigger impact on the developing critique of gender identity and power through her book, *The New Burden of Masculinity* (1957).[34] For the first time in history, men and their masculinity were getting some critical exposure.

> '*Male socialisation has become fraught with uncertainty as men are increasingly expected to show feminine traits, such as emotional expression, while maintaining their 'natural' instrumental [male] functions.*'[35]

Never before had anyone, man or woman, announced the problem of traditional masculinity and backed it up by sociological research. Seventy-five years later we are still having that discussion, though since Hacker's time it has become a global debate. Hacker, a single and divorced woman – something unacceptable in 1950s America – herself struggled against traditional gender values, both personally and professionally. She would be one of the first feminists to reify the claim that 'the personal is political'.[36]

This fresh and welcome focus on men and masculinities continued forth during the 1950s as sociologists increasingly became aware that in the West at least, times were a'changin'. As feminist sociologist Ruth Hartley predicted at the time; '*changes in women's social roles were likely to lead to feelings of anxiety, inadequacy, and hostility in men because of lack of synchronization in role-change on their part.*'[37]

---

[33] Hacker, H.M.(1951) 'Women as a Minority Group', in *Social Forces*, 30, pp. 60-69.

[34] Hacker, H.M. (1957) 'The new burdens of masculinity'; in *Marriage and Family Living*, 3, pp. 227-233.

[35] Whitehead, S.M. (2001) p.20

[36] The phrase 'the personal is political' was popularised by feminist Carol Hanisch in her 1969 essay of the same title; https://www.carolhanisch.org/CHwritings/PIP.html However, no feminist claims authorship of this phrase as it is recognised to be a defining characterisation of feminism in general.

In other words, something profound was stirring in the minds and lives of women that was not reciprocated in the minds and lives of men.

Of course, very few women or men would have read these new and original texts on gender identity. Certainly, none in my family would have ever heard of them. In the 1950s, only those benefiting from a university education in the West would have even had chance exposure to the writings of these early feminist scholars. During the 1950s, only 1.2% of American women went to college,[38] in the UK the figure was around 1%, and the vast majority of these were studying arts subjects and destined for a career in teaching.[39] But back then, few school-leavers of any gender went to university. Some 90% followed my route; leave school as soon as possible and get a job.[40]

While Hacker and Hartley in the USA were laying the foundations for feminism as practice and theory, across the pond in France a woman was building a permanent feminist monolith.

When Simone de Beauvoir's *The Second Sex* was published in 1949, I had just been born. Now, 75 years later, I recognise her book and her description of 'man as Self and woman as the Other', together with her iconic statement that 'one is not born, but becomes a woman' as the 'catalyst for challenging women's situations',[41] heralding a new understanding of gender as a social, not biological, construct. In a recent book I referred to it as a 'black swan moment' in gender relationships; a work which completely and unexpectedly forever transformed the gender political landscape.[42]

> 'During the 1950s and into the 1960s, the space of just one generation, the emergence of modern feminist thinking aligned

---

[37] Hartley, R. E. (1959) 'Sex-role pressures and the socialization of the male child', in *Psychological Reports*, 5, pp.457-468.

[38] https://sites.lib.jmu.edu/sc-interviews/2020/03/30/women-in-college-during-the-1950s/

[39] https://www.researchgate.net/figure/The-gendering-of-higher-education-in-Britain-1959-60-Source-WGPW-1962_fig3_231904466

[40] https://researchbriefings.files.parliament.uk/documents/SN04252/SN04252.pdf

[41] https://plato.stanford.edu/entries/beauvoir/#SecoSexWomaOthe

[42] Referring to the concept of 'the black swan' from philosopher, N.N.Taleb (2007) 'The Black Swan: The Impact of the Highly Improbable. London: Penguin.

with dramatic social and economic changes to produce a perfect gender storm with far-reaching implications for both women and men.'[43]

While de Beauvoir wrote one of the great feminist works, she didn't claim to be a feminist until thirty years after publication. This was because she was originally optimistic about the capacity of men to adjust to a new emancipated woman.

> 'The fact is that men are beginning to come to terms with the new condition of women; no longer feeling condemned a priori, women feel more at ease; today the working woman does not neglect her femininity, nor does she lose her sexual attraction.'[44]

In truth, *The Second Sex* is a plea to both women and men to unite, to collaborate in a just and equitable way, to value their sexual and gender differences, and to thrive together. However, she left open the door to alternative possibilities between the sexes:

> 'Her 'worlds of ideas' are not necessarily different from men's, because she will free herself by assimilating them; to know how singular she will remain and how important these singularities will continue to be, one would have to make some foolhardy predictions. What is beyond doubt is that until now women's possibilities have been stifled and lost to humanity, and in her and everyone's interests it is high time she be left to take her own chances.'[45]

Eight decades later, and it is now possible to see where women's 'assimilation of men's ideas' and their growing agency, together with men's continued resistance to emancipated females, took us. The truth is, de Beauvoir got it wrong about men but right about women; she recognised the capacity of the latter and the earth-shattering changes they would be ushering in but rather over-estimated the capacity and willingness of the former to accept and adapt to this new reality.

---

[43] Whitehead, S. (2021) p. 8

[44] de Beauvoir, S. (2015) *The Second Sex (Vintage Feminism Short Edition)*. London: Vintage. p. 52.

[45] Ibid. p.86.

The 'Swinging' Sixties

The writings of Hacker, Hartley and de Beauvoir, important as they would turn out to be, were at the time little more than stirrings of discontent; minor waves at the remotest edges of the patriarchal ocean. For most women and men nothing changed – at least in their minds, even though a lot was about to change in their lives.

By the time I reached the 1960s, the only stirrings I felt were (hetero) sexual. Masculinity was not a word I ever recall using and nor was gender. 'Sex' got used all the time. I had acquired this vague notion that men, by and large, were not to be trusted while women provided security, care and safety. Females of my generation also offered a sexual mystery so deep and powerful that I invariably froze when in their company. I readily blushed, was easily embarrassed by my sexual urges and keen to hide my constant need to masturbate. I will never forget one slightly older and more mature girlfriend informing me in 1968 and in a serious manner that I had "an inferiority complex". She was correct, though it faded away eventually. I think.

The 60s were my teenage years and I struggled through them as best I could. The only swinging I did was between my sexual imagination and my sexual reality. I remained a virgin for the first eight years of that decade and like most young men of the era lost my virginity in a clumsy fumbling rather than in a heat of passion. I was relieved to lose it. It was an essential rite of passage into adulthood, in truth into adult maleness – at least that is how I saw it. I am not sure how my girlfriend, the one who 'took' my virginity, saw it. I never asked her. We parted after ten months, the weekly sex not being enough to warrant the risk of permanence (i.e. pregnancy and marriage), which I could see looming before me like a black thunderous cloud.

The vast majority of my generation and class (working and lower-middle) never managed to avoid permanence. In my circle of friends most ended up down the aisle with the first person they slept with. Contraception was rubber and sex education – at least in my school – consisted of fearsome warnings to avoid syphilis.

I may have gone through the 60s shy, embarrassed and at times overwhelmed by my burgeoning sexuality, but growing numbers of young women and men in the USA and UK did not. Throughout this decade there was a palpable feel of cultural change in the air. It was an optimistic, vibrant and awesomely creative period. The 50s introduced us to the Brylcreemed Teddy Boys, rocking to Bill Haley and Elvis, their girlfriends in crinkly pink dresses, when along came The Beatles, The Rolling Stones, mini-skirts, free-love, pot and peace to blow that all away.

There was a brief moment, circa 1967, when I hesitate to suggest that the female prevailed in Western culture, exemplified by Woodstock, flower power, love-ins and the self-assurance of young women dancing naked to Jimi Hendrix. But it quickly died with the assassinations of Bobby Kennedy and Martin Luther King Jr, the Charles Manson murders, the Moors Murders, the My Lai massacre and the Rolling Stones' Altamont disaster. Hegemonic masculinity remained alive and well and was heralding darker days ahead.

And even those women brave or brazen enough to wear topless dresses in London's Marks and Sparks[46] mostly still yearned for romance, marriage and children. Along with the essential mortgage. Their dreams remained decidedly traditional even if their clothes were smacking traditional femininity in the face.

In a hectic decade, Western society had gone from shrewish comments over women wearing trousers in public, to mini-skirts and public nakedness. For a young man like myself, burdened by too much libido and not enough confidence, it was all rather confusing. At times it was terrifying, though it was never less than exciting.

We were indeed at the beginning of an historic revolution, the one concerned with our gender identity, though the only revolution we paid any attention to, or at least recognised as such, was that which had ushered in the Cold War, the Cuban Missile Crisis and, in the UK, had served to expose the John Profumo affair and the dallying of his 'girlfriends', Mandy Rice-Davies and Christine Keeler.[47]

Although critical gender discourse was starting to percolate from the feminist theoreticians in universities through to the masses, it was nothing more than a slow trickle. Indeed, as far as most academics were concerned, feminism was very much a side-show to the 'main event', which in those days was Marxism. This heavily structural theory, blessed by male philosophers such as Althusser, Gramsci and Marcuse, ruled in universities, not as practice but certainly as theory. This was still the case thirty years later when I landed a lectureship in Education at Keele University, UK.

---

[46] Marks and Spencer – the iconic UK High Street retailer founded in 1884

[47] I am referring here to the Russian revolution of the early 20th century. https://www.theguardian.com/uk-news/2020/jan/04/profumo-scandal-trial-of-christine-keeler-bbc

But none of that mattered to me back then. No thought of further or higher education ever entered my head. I had no qualifications and didn't need them. Like all my male friends, I just wanted a steady job, a bit of spare cash, a nice car and, eventually a home with wife and child(ren). Nothing too ambitious really, though looking back I can see how fortunate I was just to even have such aspirations.

Not that there was a lack of revolutionaries if one cared to look, and I am not referring to those who sang so compellingly about revolution such as Pete Seeger, Joan Baez and Bob Dylan. Oxbridge in particular was proving a fertile ground for the furtherance of 'feminist fundamentalism', aptly demonstrated by Rose Dugdale (eventually to graduate as an IRA terrorist and bomber), and Jenny Grove storming the bastions of male entitlement by demanding to join the all-male Oxford Union Society. They won that battle but had to gate-crash the Union in male disguise to do so. Although this historic event has gone largely unnoticed in the current 'gender wars', one historian has described it as a 'huge victory [for women's rights] which changed British establishment politics for ever'.[48]

If first-wave feminist activism began in the early 1900s with its focus primarily on women's suffrage, it wasn't until the 1960s and the emergence of second-wave feminism that it became a 'movement'.[49] In the USA, civil rights issues and the Vietnam War were galvanising a younger generation to challenge the powers that be. Campuses became hotbeds of protest by an eclectic mix of youthful social reformers – black power militants, anti-capitalists, anti-war marchers, and gay rights activists – while feminist became a badge that many young Americans, at least those at college, were proud to wear.

Reinforced by a fast-growing literary accompaniment to second-wave feminism, espousing the grand and worthy aims of a new gender order and persuasively articulated by the likes of Gloria Steinem, Betty Friedan and Mary Daly, feminists found their voice and confidence to challenge patriarchy in all its varied forms. And they had much success especially in equal employment legislation, reproductive rights, raising awareness

---

[48] O'Driscoll, S. (2022) *Heiress, Rebel, Vigilante, Bomber: The Extraordinary Life of Rose Dugdale*. London: Penguin. P.35.

[49] https://www.gale.com/primary-sources/womens-studies/collections/second-wave-feminism#:~:text=Second%20Wave%20Feminism%3A%20Collections,spread%20to%20other%20Western%20countries.

around domestic abuse[50] and in exposing the flaws in the 'perfect American nuclear family',[51] now under serious threat from 'disorganised capitalism',[52] an emerging global economy, and fast-developing post-industrialisation.[53]

However, no matter the avidly determined and enthusiastic outpourings of feminists on US and UK campuses, I was never convinced of the loyalty of their male comrades. It seemed to me, and still does, that those young, fresh-faced beauties in mini-skirts and little else attracted male comrades not so much for the freedom of women but for the free love from women.

For most men, even radicalised students, when push came to shove, sex invariably trumped politics. And thus far, apart from some notable radical feminist texts from the likes of Mary Daly, attributed as saying…

> *"If life is to survive on this planet, there must be a decontamination of the Earth. I think this will be accompanied by an evolutionary process that will result in a drastic reduction in the population of males."*[54]

…most men were hardly in danger of being personally challenged by this particular revolution. They continued to inhabit a mental bubble which acquired its security and certainties from a decidedly traditional masculinity.

Compulsory heterosexuality and its attendant outlets such as *Playboy* magazine and the Playboy Club (where feminist Gloria Steinem went undercover to expose the male chauvinism of its clientele), defined America during this era as much if not more than 'The Feminist Mystique',[55] with *Playboy* magazine peaking at seven million copies a month by the early 1970s. While back in my home town of Southport, if I wasn't reading *Playboy* I could always pop along to the summer 'beauty contests' long held on Southport promenade. No, I never attended – they offered a decidedly

---

[50] https://www.gale.com/primary-sources/womens-studies/collections/second-wave-feminism   https://www.humanrightscareers.com/issues/second-wave-feminism-history-main-ideas-impact/

[51] https://dumas.ccsd.cnrs.fr/dumas-00680821/document

[52] Lash, S. and Urry, J. (1987) *The End of Organised Capitalism*. Cambridge: Polity.

[53] Bell, D. (1976) *The Coming of Post-Industrial Society. A Venture in Social Forecasting*. New York: Basic Books.

[54] Quoted in Whitehead, S. (2021). P. 9.

[55] Friedan, B. (1963) *The Feminine Mystique*. New York: Norton

50s' vision of feminine beauty and anyway, I was far too busy playing the guitar.

At this point it's important to distinguish between the 60s' sexual revolution and the 60s' gender revolution. These two overlapped but were certainly not the same thing. The former was about having more sex without guilt or shame, while the latter was determined to change a whole world order. Like pretty much every other male, I too felt more attached to the sex one than the gender one. Indeed, for the most part the gender (aka feminist) revolution totally passed me by. I was vaguely aware that there were women rising up who called themselves feminists, but they didn't live near me and I never came across them in the pubs and clubs on Merseyside. The feminists appeared to hang out in universities and I'd never been near a university and had no plans to do so. The sex revolution was a whole lot closer, literally and emotionally. All my friends were having sex and several had to get married due to unplanned pregnancies. I eventually caught up with the trend – sex not pregnancy – but as I say, it took me a little longer.

But were the girls that interested in sex? It seems unlikely. When nineteen-year-old Cathy McGowan, the trendy presenter of Rediffusion's new youth culture TV pop show, *Ready, Steady, Go!* was asked what mattered most to teenagers – sex, music or fashion – she unerringly answered "Fashion".[56]

And were the working-class, or even middle-class, teenage girls interested in feminism? Hardly. What they were interested in was a man who had a regular job, then marriage and children – in that order. Even in the 'swinging' sixties no teenage girl wanted to end up pregnant and unmarried. No teenage lad, for that matter.

For most young women during the 60s, even if they took the time to think about a gender (feminist) revolution, what it likely meant for them was being free to dance naked in a field at the Isle of Wight festival or to go and live in San Francisco with the flower-power people and 'drop out'.

However, while that may appear frivolous or even hedonistic, it does reveal the connection between the sex and gender revolutions: women's bodies.

At the start of the twentieth century, women didn't own very much at all and certainly not control over their bodies, their fertility nor their sexuality. Patriarchy was firmly established through law, religion and culture, leaving women free to do, well, very little. Only the very wealthy women had some respite, though even they could only exercise power as

---

[56] Kynstan, D. (2023) *A Northern Wind. Britain 1962-65*. London: Bloomsbury. P. 300

proxy if they had truly powerful and wealthy husbands. The 1960s' sexual revolution shook up this structural arrangement. Women in the USA and UK were freer to express their sexuality (my mother bought a copy of *Lady Chatterley's Lover*, banned until 1960); they could stay single if they chose (fear of spinsterhood was declining); divorce, separation and cohabitation steadily became more socially acceptable; university attendance was rising for women and so were the job opportunities; while abortion was legalised in the UK in 1968 and eleven US states liberalised their abortion laws at the end of the decade. The so-called 'permissive society'[57] was further fuelled by the contraceptive pill, introduced in the US and UK at the start of the 60s though initially restricted to married women. As far as the 'freeing up' of women's bodies, the sexual freedom proffered during the 1960s was an important, albeit hesitant, step towards feminism.

The globalising energy of the 1960s generated a counter-culture based on the promotion and privileging of youthful creativity, notably through the arts and music, reinforced by political awareness of and active resistance to the Vietnam War, racism, colonialism, nuclear armament, and capitalism. This was evidenced by mass demonstrations across the USA, and in London, Paris, Amsterdam and Berlin. Was this part of second-wave feminist activism? Yes, but only a part. Women of all ages participated in these protests, on campus and off, thereby providing them with a hardening political awareness and confident activism which was itself globalising – by the end of the 60s over thirty countries had feminist movements[58] – but while there was a lot of shouting about freedom, justice, equality and peace, few men were listening. There is little evidence that men took this counter culture as a signal to change their masculinity, become more enlightened as males and adopt a more progressive way of being.

In short, while the 60s provided sexual freedoms, great music, protest and revolutionary slogans, and created a feminist consciousness in a great many women around the world, feminism still faced a long road ahead.

---

[57] https://britishonlinearchives.com/posts/category/contextual-essays/484/the-transforming-effect-of-the-1960s. Collins. M. (2007) *The Permissive Society and its Enemies: Sixties British Culture.* London: Rivers Oram Press.

[58] https://projects.iq.harvard.edu/files/soc_fem/files/de_haan_2018_global_left-feminist_1960s.pdf

The Dark, Dangerous, Dividing Seventies

On 4th May 1970, the Ohio National Guard fired on a crowd of Kent State University protesters, killing four students and wounded nine others, all unarmed. On that day, the 'swinging sixties' came to an abrupt and violent end.[59]

I barely remember it. Because I was in love. I floated through 1970 on a cloud of romance and sexual discovery, reaching my majority in the August (aged twenty-one) blissfully happy and completely enwrapped in monogamy. I walked down the aisle in February 1971, a callow youth with a big grin on his face and a beautiful bride by his side.

My wife Rosemary (aged twenty-one) and I moved into a new home, bought on a manageable mortgage, and settled down to domestic life. We quickly acquired a dog. Half a century later, such a lifestyle for twenty-one-year-olds would look decidedly odd. But back then, twenty-one-year-olds got married all the time. Over the next two years, my wife and I would attend another six weddings; two cousins, three friends, and my sister. All were aged under twenty-four. My sister was aged eighteen, her husband, nineteen. Within a few years, five of these marriages had produced children. Although there wasn't a declared feminist among the wives, this generation of women would help contribute to the fast-looming gender revolution.

The 70s weren't merely the decade during which I and my friends (and wife) came of age, it was the decade that feminism came of age. The UK had the Women's Liberation Movement[60] demanding not just equality but massive social and gender transformation, while the USA had the National Organization for Women; 'their eschatological aim to topple the patriarchal system in which men by birth-right control all of society's levers of power – in government, industry, education, science, the arts'.[61] Feminism was going global by the early 1970s, impacting not across the Global North but increasingly the Global South.[62]

There was a new and strident radicalism to 70s feminism that wasn't apparent in the 60s. It spawned 'radical feminist theory' and was captured most powerfully in the remarkable book, *Sexual Politics* by Kate Millett (it

---

[59] https://www.kent.edu/may-4-historical-accuracy

[60] https://journals.openedition.org/rfcb/1688

[61] https://edition.cnn.com/2015/07/22/living/the-seventies-feminism-womens-lib/index.html

[62] https://www.sciencedirect.com/science/article/pii/S0277539523001085

was her PhD thesis).[63] I was still drawing on Millett's theories twenty years later when I did my MA in Sociology. As one American male professor put it:

> "Reading [Sexual Politics] is like sitting with your testicles in a nutcracker"[64]

And he was right. Feminism was now getting into top gear and that meant hitting men where it hurt – in their masculine entitlement.

Another feminist getting into full flight was Gloria Steinem, who in 1969 had written a *New York Magazine* article, 'After Black Power, Women's Liberation'.[65] A year later, in an evaluation of women's liberation progress, she wrote the following:

> 'In Women's Lib Utopia, there will be free access to good jobs – and decent pay for the bad ones women have been performing all along, including housework… Schools and universities will help break down traditional sex roles, even when parents will not. Half the teachers will be men, a rarity now at preschool and elementary levels: girls will not necessarily serve cookies or boys hoist the flag.'[66]

During the early 1970s, there was a definite anger and frustration in feminist writings, and an increasingly accusatory finger being pointed at men, misogyny and institutionalised sexism. This was no more powerfully demonstrated than in the writings of Andrea Dworkin.

If you were a man who wanted to stereotype feminists as American, overweight, dungaree-wearing, angry, and as tough as hell on men, then you need look no further than Ms Dworkin. She certainly scared me. But that was back in my ignorant youth. Today I find myself drawing ever closer to Dworkin's unvarnished truth about men. Here are some examples:

---

[63] Millet, K. (1970) *Sexual Politics*. Garden City, NY: Doubleday. For an early elaboration of radical feminism see Tong, R. (1994) *Feminist Thought*. London: Routledge. For a more recent analysis, see Tong, R. and Botts, F.T. (2024) *Feminist Thought: A More Comprehensive Introduction*. London: Routledge.

[64] https://edition.cnn.com/2015/07/22/living/the-seventies-feminism-womens-lib/index.html https://www.tandfonline.com/doi/full/10.1080/09612025.2023.2277488

[65] https://nymag.com/news/politics/46802/

[66] https://time.com/5795657/gloria-steinem-womens-liberation-progress/

> 'Feminism is hated because women are hated. Anti-feminism is a direct expression of misogyny; it is the political defense of women hating'
>
> 'Men are distinguished from women by their commitment to do violence rather than be victimized by it.'
>
> 'Only when manhood is dead – and it will perish when ravaged femininity no longer sustains it – only then will we know what it is to be free.'[67]

She never said "*all men are rapists, and that's all they are*" – that was her radical feminist colleague, Marilyn French. But she might well have done.[68]

Over a three-decade period I have experienced a number of feminist transitions, at least as a pro-feminist man. I began with liberal feminism (like many do), took up with feminist poststructuralism because quite frankly it is the only sociological theory that explains gender identity, but, like many other feminists, I am now gravitating towards radical feminism, attracted by the sheer conviction, force and accuracy of its statements.[69]

Is it possible for a man to be a radical feminist? Well, I guess Dworkin's long-time male partner John Stoltenberg managed it, otherwise I cannot see him lasting long with Andrea – they were together 31 years.[70] In which case, perhaps I can too. Though it helps being in my mid-seventies and with no sexual desire left whatsoever and therefore no chance of getting my political and heterosexual 'interests' confused.

While the radical feminists of the early 1970s could be seen as gate-crashing the historical patriarchal party and kicking over the tables, their theory drew heavily on women as the 'Other', the concept originally devised by de Beauvoir twenty years previously; and de Beauvoir certainly wasn't a radical, at least not when she wrote *The Second Sex*. In truth, all

---

[67] https://www.goodreads.com/author/quotes/23879.Andrea_Dworkin

[68] https://en.wikipedia.org/wiki/Andrea_Dworkin   https://en.wikipedia.org/wiki/Marilyn_French

[69] https://www.theguardian.com/lifeandstyle/2019/apr/16/why-andrea-dworkin-is-the-radical-visionary-feminist-we-need-in-our-terrible-times   https://jwa.org/encyclopedia/article/dworkin-andrea

[70] https://www.feminist.com/resources/artspeech/genwom/andreadworkin.html
https://www.theguardian.com/books/2025/feb/23/andrea-dworkins-women-hating-pornography-right-wing-john-stoltenberg?CMP=Share_iOSApp_Other

feminist theories, and there a now a number of them, owe allegiance to de Beauvoir because she was the first to clearly declare that women (and by implication, men) are not biological entities but social beings. But what the radical feminists achieved was a powerful resistance to male power and its expression as rape, abuse or violence against women. And as the gender revolution has evolved I find increasing numbers of women returning to the concepts espoused by Mary Daly, Andrea Dworkin, Kate Millet, Marilyn French and Shulamith Firestone.[71] One can read radical feminism in the statements of women around the world today – I read them daily on LinkedIn. Many of these women may not realise they are voicing an anger and protest which goes back to the 1970s, but they are.

While the feminists around the world, and most definitely in the USA, Germany, Australia and the UK, were attacking patriarchal structures, practices and attitudes, I was pulling pints of beer in a hotel in Leeds city centre. In 1975, Rosemary and I, along with our twelve-month-old son, had quit sunny Southport for darker Leeds, beginning our journey into hotel and restaurant management. Leeds was dark for a number of reasons; not just the soot and grime of the Victorian back-to-back houses and majestic Town Hall. Three months after we arrived and took up our assistant management post at the Guildford Hotel, Leeds, (October, 1975) a 28-year-old mother of four and apparent sex-worker, Wilma McGann, was found brutally murdered in the Chapeltown area of Leeds. This was the first of thirteen officially recorded killings by the man who would go on to achieve infamy as the Yorkshire Ripper.

Reclaiming the Night

Over the past seven decades I have noticed how individual male behaviour can act as a dramatic catalyst on women, angering them to such an extent that they rise up as a group with a hitherto unleashed power, thereby pushing the gender revolution irrevocably forward.[72] To be sure, the anger

---

[71] Tong, R. (1994)

[72] Another prominent example being the kidnapping, rape and murder of Sara Everard, 2021 (UK). Examples at time of writing; Giselle Pelicot mass rape case (France); Conan McGregor civil rape case (Ireland); Doctor's rape and murder in Kolkata (India); mass stabbing and killing of women in Bondi, Sydney (Australia); spate of femicides (Kenya); murder of Giulia Cecchettin by her ex-boyfriend, Venice (Italy); murder of BBC racing commentator, John Hunt's, wife and two daughters by Kyle Clifford, the younger daughter's former partner (UK);

settles down afterwards – no more street protests, for example – but it never entirely goes away. The catalyst, whatever/whoever it is, remains in the consciousness of women, probably for their lifetimes. The most obvious example is the global #MeToo Movement and Harvey Weinstein, discussed below and in Chapter 3, but long before then, in 1976, Peter Sutcliffe (aka The Yorkshire Ripper), triggered a similar outpouring of rage from women across the UK and especially in Yorkshire, where Sutcliffe mostly conducted his murderous rampage against women.[73]

For me, this dark episode was also a catalyst of sorts, because I was close to the 'action'. Not only was I living in Leeds during this period, but by August 1976, Rosemary and I were landlords/managers of The Jubilee pub, wine bar, and restaurant, situated exactly opposite Leeds Town Hall, the Law Courts, and close to West Yorkshire Police HQ. Judges, lawyers, solicitors and especially detectives were my regular customers. Many no doubt came to my bars to drown their sorrows, because from 1976 to when Sutcliffe was caught on 2nd January 1981, the West Yorkshire Police force was subject to the most intense national scrutiny and criticism, not only over its incompetent handling of the 'Ripper Case' but especially its institutionalised sexism, misogyny and tendency to stereotype most of Sutcliffe's victims as prostitutes. The gender most angry at all this was, predictably, the female one.[74]

The first 'reclaim the night' protest took place in Leeds on 12th November 1977. This and future marches, mostly by women, charged and changed the atmosphere between women and men, and between women and the police. While few, if any, men felt personally threatened by a crazed misogynistic serial killer loose on the streets, every woman in Yorkshire, indeed across the north of England, certainly did. One of the most telling points of the protesting women was that while the West Yorkshire police had advised women not to go out at night, no such advice was given to men.

Execution in Japan of Takahiro Shiraishi (dubbed the 'Twitter Killer') for the murder of eight women and one man during 2017.

[73] https://en.wikipedia.org/wiki/Peter_Sutcliffe Cook, C. (2024) *Peter Sutcliffe: The Full Crimes of the Yorkshire Ripper.* Barnsley, UK: Pen and Sword Books

[74] https://www.theguardian.com/uk-news/2020/nov/13/it-was-toxic-how-sexism-threw-police-off-the-trail-of-the-yorkshire-ripper   https://historyinpolitics.org/2021/06/19/the-yorkshire-ripper-investigation-a-total-disaster-from-a-feminist-perspective/

> *"That was what partly fuelled our anger and rage, that in effect there was a curfew on women but not on men."*[75]

The Leeds organisers of 'reclaim the night' were inspired by the first recorded march against male violence, held in Brussels in 1976. Since then, marches and rallies by women (and men) protesting male violence against women and femicide, have become a global phenomenon, occurring in, for example, Mexico, Australia, Spain, Ireland, France, UK, USA, Bangladesh, India, Kenya, Bosnia and Herzegovina, Cameroon, Hungary, Kosovo, Kyrgyzstan, Pakistan, Turkey, Iran, Egypt, Peru and Liberia.[76] At the time of writing, the first march in the Ivory Coast against femicide has just taken place[77] while the 'Million Women Rise' international march was held on 8th March 2025.[78]

Neither Rosemary nor I joined those historic the Leeds protesters; neither of us were rally-goers even though we certainly had a lot of first-hand evidence of the sexist attitudes of the 1970s West Yorkshire police force. Nor were we declared feminists: indeed, like most of our generation, 'feminist' was a term we couldn't readily associate with even while we supported and largely lived out its the core values of equality of opportunity. In that respect, we were no different to a great many British twenty-somethings who'd not had the benefit of a university education; aware but not yet totally awake.

But growing numbers of young people certainly were awake. The 70s was an intoxicating time to be a feminist, attracting women of all races, classes, backgrounds and political beliefs. In a multitude of ways, from advancing feminist theory to attacking institutionalised sexism, from protest marches against male violence to instigating Equal Opportunity legislation,[79] the

---

[75] https://mancunion.com/2022/03/20/the-origins-and-history-of-reclaim-the-night/

[76] https://www.researchgate.net/publication/304802105_From_Brussels_to_Leeds_San_Francisco_Delhi_The_global_march_of_Reclaim_the_Night https://www.aljazeera.com/gallery/2024/11/26/thousands-rally-across-the-world-calling-for-end-to-violence-against-women https://lens.civicus.org/from-outrage-to-action-2024s-global-protests-against-gender-based-violence/

[77] https://www.theguardian.com/global-development/2024/dec/20/ivorian-women-girls-femicide-ivory-coast-march-grand-bassam

[78] https://www.millionwomenrise.com/

[79] https://www.eeoc.gov/history/eeoc-history-1970-1979 https://www.legislation.gov.uk/ukpga/1970/41/enacted

seventies decade is when feminism went from being a 'side show' to entering the main political arena.

Thatcher's Eighties

It's tempting to describe the 'rise of women' as an untroubled linear process but that is far from being accurate; linear and progressive its history might be, untroubled it certainly was not. And too often feminism's strongest opponents have come from within the 'sisterhood' itself. The American feminists had Phyllis Stewart Schlafly to contend with, an American attorney, conservative activist, anti-feminist, anti-abortionist who was vehemently opposed to gay rights.[80] The UK had Margaret Thatcher, one of the most anti-feminist British women of the decade but also the most powerful; the first woman leader of the Conservative Party and first woman to be elected (in May 1979) British Prime Minister. Thatcher was the ultimate feminist enigma: a confident, powerful woman who dominated the many old-school entitled male politicians around her; a proud 'Iron Lady', who was feminist in her independent attitude and dismissal of 'weak' and 'egotistical' men but certainly no promoter of the sisterhood. Looking back, this makes me wonder what on earth I was thinking when I joined the Conservative Party in August 1985, and shortly afterwards stood for election as a Leeds City Councillor.

I began the 80s as landlord of the Woodside Tavern, a delightfully profitable pub and restaurant in leafy Horsforth, north Leeds. I and my family had thankfully left behind the tough city centre. The job was so comfortable that it was boring and I quickly looked for other outlets for my energy. Politics came to mind, though as any pub landlord will testify, it's wise never to get into politics. Nevertheless, that is where I headed. Not that I was a natural Conservative. At the previous General Election, I'd voted Independent and was one of the few people I knew who opposed the Falklands War. But I did like the idea of representing Horsforth as a Councillor and the local Conservatives welcomed me in.

By 1985 I was far from being a feminist or even concerned with gender politics. I certainly wasn't going to stand on any feminist platform, not least because it would have been political suicide. I stood for Thatcherism – as that was expected of me, even while I didn't fully understand or appreciate what Thatcherism meant in reality. My brief but most interesting excursion into local politics came to its natural end in 1989, and I was not displeased

---

[80] https://www.history.com/news/equal-rights-amendment-failure-phyllis-schlafly

about that. But while I was busying myself trying to become a Leeds City Councillor (I failed), feminists around the world had their own battles, notably 'fighting the backlash'.[81]

During the 1980s, Thatcher and her political soulmate in the USA, President Ronald Reagan,[82] aided and abetted by a collapsing Soviet Union, introduced a new right, conservative arrogance to Western politics that over forty years on is still with us, but which has since morphed into a harsher, illiberal, anti-immigration, isolationist, anti-feminist, anti-LGBTQ+ movement, behind which are trooping growing numbers of men. This has now become a contributing aspect of the gender divergence discussed in Chapter 5. None of this was foreseen by feminists in the 80s: they were more concerned with trying to survive because feminist had become a dirty word, especially among young women.

> "In the 1980s, feminism was out of fashion with most young women. Like flappers in the 1920s, these women looked upon feminists of the previous decade as old hat, stodgy, and unpleasantly angry."[83]

> "[In the 1980s]... taking a stand on anything remotely construed as a women's issue aroused strange and strong suspicions." ibid

> "During our 'coming of age' years from 1980 to 1990, young feminists didn't seem to exist," ibid

> "For a great many young women in the 80s, 'feminist' conjured up 'caricatures of bra-burning, hairy-legged, Amazon, castrating, militant-almost-anti-feminine women." ibid

> "We [feminists] watched as the whole neo-liberal structure swept us off the table... the media completely turned its back on us as they danced to the new-liberal tune."[84]

---

[81] https://www.cambridge.org/core/books/abs/womens-movement-against-sexual-harassment/fighting-the-backlash-feminist-activism-in-the-1980s/B8E4AE9F64437C1CE62B6B4AADC9685F

[82] https://picturethis.museumca.org/timeline/reagan-years-1980s/womens-rights/info

[83] https://academic.oup.com/book/47562/chapter-abstract/422321165?redirectedFrom=fulltext

[84] https://www.financialjustice.ie/econowha1/econo-wha-blog-posts/2b-being-a-feminist-in-the-1980s/

While most people I socialised with in the 80s professed to loathe Ronald Reagan and Margaret Thatcher and all they stood for, I suspect many secretly admired them. People certainly voted for them in large numbers. And a key element in this attraction was the sense of possibility that these two politicians offered to 'ordinary folk'. Despite the harshness of new right politics, the implicit racism in much of the new right rhetoric, performance-driven managerialist work cultures, and the unforgiving liberal market economy, one underlying theme both in the USA and UK politics during this decade was 'independence', usually floated alongside 'entrepreneurship'. People were encouraged to be independent and strive for themselves; it was a cornerstone of Thatcherism. When Thatcher claimed "there is no such thing as society, only the individual" not only did she mean it but her words spoke directly to the aspirations of millions of young people now coming out of universities and heading into work.

Of course, many voters did loathe Thatcher: the miners, the teachers, the intellectuals and, ironically, the British aristocracy, especially. But love her or loathe her, Thatcher's creed wriggled itself into the minds of a younger generation seeking a more materially enriched, individualistic, agentic life and took root. While Thatcherism left little room for feminism as an identity in the minds of ordinary women, in one important respect it didn't matter. *Because Thatcher's creed already contained the DNA of feminism* through its declaration and promotion of feminine power and agency, ironically exemplified by a woman who loathed feminists and was understandably loathed by them.

So, despite Thatcher's best efforts, feminism didn't disappear during the 80s; it just lingered underground waiting for the frost to disappear and environmental conditions to improve. The women weren't out on the street like they'd been in the 70s, but the core element of feminism – women doing it for themselves – was very much alive, perhaps more alive and well than ever in human history. And one place this was particularly apparent was the academy: universities, which is where I eventually met up with feminism in the early 1990s as a postgraduate student. This is when I met my first (academic) feminists face-to-face and discovered I was not the man I thought I was.

Chapter 3: Independent Femininity

As a politicised identity that a majority of women would enthusiastically embrace and own, feminism didn't exactly die in the 80s but it did become marginalised and unfashionable. Feminism got weaker as a core identity around which women would align, though got stronger in terms of its diversity and inclusivity, for example seeing the emergence of black feminism/feminists, feminist community projects, ecofeminism/feminists, and Latino feminism/feminists.[85]

It was no surprise that one of the most popular feminist books of this era was *Backlash* by Susan Faludi (1991) in which she examined the 'undeclared war against American women', the rise of the anti-abortion movement, increases in male harassment of women and political/social pushbacks against equal rights for women.[86]

Yet despite the growing resistance to feminism/feminists by the new right and conservative/religious groups, in respect of its influence feminism

---

[85] See, for examples and discussion, 'Black Feminism in the 1980ss' https://www.jstor.org/stable/43824458; 'Black Feminist Thought' https://negrasoulblog.wordpress.com/wp-content/uploads/2016/04/patricia-hill-collins-black-feminist-thought.pdf; https://nmaahc.si.edu/explore/stories/revolutionary-practice-black-feminisms; https://www.vice.com/en/article/revisiting-michele-wallaces-essential-black-feminist-text-black-macho-2/; https://womenslibrary.org.uk/2021/08/17/feminist-housing-activism-in-the-1970s-1980s-1-making-space-for-feminist-infrastructures/; https://www.financialjustice.ie/econowha1/econo-wha-blog-posts/2b-being-a-feminist-in-the-1980s/; https://www.bbc.com/news/articles/cn7me4688yno; https://ehne.fr/en/encyclopedia/themes/ecology-and-environment/gender-and-environment/ecofeminism-in-europe-a-social-movement-1980s; https://www.jstor.org/stable/43247551; https://theconversation.com/how-latin-american-feminists-shifted-global-understanding-of-gender-based-violence-173121; https://academic.oup.com/edited-volume/34259/chapter/290462295; The Development of Chicana Feminist Discourse, 1970-1980, https://www.jstor.org/stable/189983

[86] Faludi, S. (1991) *Backlash: The Undeclared War Against American Women*. New York: Crown.

not only survived being 'unfashionable' but went on to live in the minds of women everywhere. And its greatest and most lasting legacy is the critical contribution it made to the creation of independent femininity; a powerful and assertive way of being female which women of all types are now confidently performing in every corner of the globe. As I explain in this chapter, while feminist remains a difficult and controversial identity for most women, it is undoubtedly the mother of independent femininity, largely marginalising hegemonic/traditional femininity.

From Feminism to Independent Femininity

Over the years I have lost count of how many women have replied to my question; "are you a feminist?" by answering: "No, I don't hate men". For years I have had that exact or very similar response from women around the world, not just in the UK and USA. This leaves me no longer surprised or disappointed when a woman who, in every aspect of her being, expresses a feminist identity, claims not to be a feminist. Of course, this is not true of all women, but certainly the majority. This is supported by research which shows that only 29% of American women identify as feminist and only 34% of British women.[87] A global study of 31 mostly high- and upper-income countries revealed that 39% of women identified as feminist. Only two countries, India and Spain, had a majority of women who saw themselves as feminist.[88] While such surveys can show slightly different results over time, there is no question that feminism has not achieved one of its original objectives: to become a globalised political standpoint for the majority of women.

In this regard, the anti-feminists of the 80s and 90s certainly achieved their aim in denigrating feminism and making it a negative label for most women. I have laid the 'blame' for this largely at the door of Margaret Thatcher at least in the UK context, but maybe the feminists of the 70s were just too strident for a public still wrapped up in traditional gender values and identities? One cannot blame 80s' Thatcherism for the fact that a millennial woman in today's Brazil, Vietnam, Italy or Thailand is rejecting feminism not least because she associates it with men-hating radicalised women. But whatever the reasons, and one can endlessly speculate on the

---

[87] https://www.reddit.com/r/AskFeminists/comments/hjh58t/only_29_of_american_women_identify_as_feminists/?rdt=36610

[88] https://www.statista.com/chart/32523/agreement-with-statement-i-define-myself-as-a-feminist/

causes and deduce any number of alternative influences, the fact remains that feminism as a political movement took severe blows in the 80s from which, to date, it has only partially recovered.

And yet these same women who are today denying the feminist label will espouse a way of being a woman which is entirely feminist: independent, agentic, assertive, self-actualising and in no way accepting of male dominance and traditional gender values.[89] This strongly suggests that women around the world are the 'daughters' of the feminists of the 70s, 80s and 90s, even if they don't realise it or want to realise it. What this tells us is that the discourses defining a core feminism never really went away, even if 'feminist' is no longer a banner behind which a majority of women will flock to march.

The great strength of feminism is also its great weakness: its identity-validating properties. This means that once a woman has declared herself to be a feminist, then it is an identity label likely to remain with her for life – and for the majority of women, feminist is not an identity they seek for themselves. Recall de Beauvoir claiming not to be a feminist, even after having written the definitive feminist text of the twentieth century. Why? Because she still had hope of the continuation and improvement of the male-female relationship dynamic. Eventually, de Beauvoir gave up her resistance to the feminist identity and embraced it, in so doing effectively declaring the end of her optimism in men's capacity or willingness to change. She never doubted what women with a feminist mindset could achieve – a dramatic shift in the traditional gender arrangement – which is where we are today.

What has replaced feminism as a political gender identity for a majority of women is something much more powerful and more durable, but also a lot less politically contentious: independent femininity. In its progression into the minds and hearts of millions of young and older women around the world, independent femininity has not only marginalised traditional, hegemonic ways of being a woman, exemplified as traditional femininity and defined below, but directly challenged men and traditional masculinity.

Today, it is independent femininity that is the real threat to those men holding on to traditional masculinity, not feminism. And unlike feminism/feminists – an easy target for the incels, the male fundamentalists and the misogynists who often degrade them as 'feminazis' – it is almost impossible

---

[89] An iconic example of a woman presenting simultaneously both a 'non-feminist, pro-female independence' conundrum is Lady Gaga. https://msmagazine.com/2010/03/11/is-lady-gaga-a-feminist-or-isnt-she/; https://www.theguardian.com/music/2010/sep/17/lady-gaga-feminist-icon

to hit at and degrade independent femininity. Why? Because it is not a political identity supported by an ideology but simply a way of being an aspirational woman in the twenty-first century. You can be a woman with independent femininity and all that entails, without hating men; you can even love a few of them.

There remains, however, an interesting question to address. How exactly did feminism manage to survive Thatcherism and Reaganism, the two free-market ideologies that at least in part it challenged? A large part of that answer lies within the academic profession.

The University Feminists

As a declared feminist male, I am in a very small minority, which is fine because for me feminism and its theories are more than a political standpoint; they have helped me understand identity, especially men and masculinities, and consequently my self. But then I have long been part of the sociological feminist academy; the university brigade who spend much of their time researching and writing about gender, sex and sexuality. I've been doing precisely that for over thirty years, so feminist is not only my personal label but also my academic and professional identity. And it began to be so in 1991.

My introduction to feminism and feminist theory was on my MA course in Leisure and Work at Leeds Metropolitan University. Feminist Theory was a second-year option module I could easily have avoided but which I opted for, despite being initially very hesitant. I knew this module would challenge me personally and I was not sure I wanted to be challenged about my attitudes towards women and feminism. I was aged 42, in my second marriage, a father, and several years into my new career as a college lecturer in leisure, sport and tourism – I felt comfortable in myself as a man, though that 'comfort' (as I soon discovered) was founded on stereotypes, illusion, myth and fear.

The director of the MA course was a feminist, Professor Sheila Scraton.[90] The Head of Department was a feminist: Professor Margaret Talbot.[91] And

---

[90] Sheila is an internationally recognised expert on gender and physical education. She went on to become Pro Vice Chancellor and Director of University Research at Leeds Beckett University until her retirement in 2008. https://books.google.co.th/books/about/Shaping_Up_to_Womanhood.html?id=Ve-1AAAAIAAJ&redir_esc=y

several of the lecturers were feminists, both women and men.[92] For these intellectuals, and many like them around the world, feminism may have taken a battering from Thatcherism, Reaganism and the New Right, but they were in for the long haul. They astutely realised that the New Right could not stand in the way of history and they recognised the direction of gender history in particular: it wasn't going backwards.

As it transpired, my timing couldn't have been more perfect for being introduced to feminism; 1990 witnessed the start of a new and very exciting Third Wave in feminist theory, sparked by American philosopher Judith Butler and her landmark book, *Gender Trouble* (1990).[93] This work, introducing and defining feminist poststructuralism (which I summarised in Chapter 1), had a very similar impact to de Beauvoir's *The Second Sex*, published forty years earlier. Some 35 years on and Butler is still providing feminists and philosophers with cutting-edge enquiry into gender and identity.[94]

I have detailed and defined the first, second and third waves of feminist theory in a previously published book[95] so I won't repeat that here, though it is useful to understand that by the 1990s feminist theories had multiplied.

---

[91] Professor Margaret Talbot OBE (1946-2014) was President of the International Association of Physical Education for Girls and Women from 1997 to 2005. She was Carnegie Research Professor at Leeds Metropolitan University where she was also Head of Sport. https://www.sportanddev.org/latest/news/margaret-talbot-champion-universal-access-physical-education-and-sport

[92] One example being Dr Peter Bramham, Senior Lecturer in Leisure Studies when I was studying at LMU. Peter was a big influence on my early learning and critical awareness of sociological issues especially around race, class, gender and nationality. See, Bramham, P. and Wagg, S. (eds) (2014) *An Introduction to Leisure Studies: Principals and Practices*. London: Sage.

[93] Butler, J. (1990) *Gender Trouble*. New York: Routledge. Also, Butler, J. (1993) *Bodies That Matter: The Discursive Limits of 'Sex'*. New York: Routledge. Note that feminist poststructuralist theory as developed by Judith Butler draws heavily on the writings and theories of, amongst others, Michel Foucault. See Whitehead, S, Talahite, A. and Moodley, R. (2013) *Gender and Identity: Key Themes and New Directions*, Oxford: Oxford University Press, for introduction.

[94] At time of writing, Judith Butler's most recent book is 'Who's Afraid of Gender?', (2024) London: Penguin.

[95] Whitehead, Talahite and Moodley, (2013)

They included, for example, Liberal Feminism, Marxist Feminism, Socialist Feminism, Radical Feminism, Psychoanalytical Feminism and Postmodern Feminism.[96] Globally, a growing number of universities were drawing on these diverse theories to understand changes in male and female identities, powers, subjectivities and experiences. Feminist theories were increasingly being used to examine everything from nursing to politics, architecture to engineering. Concurrent to these intellectual advancements, male feminists were also slowly emerging in universities where they were focused on studying men and masculinities – very soon I'd become one of them.

This intellectualised feminist explosion can be easily overlooked when examining the rise of women over the past seventy years and the emergence of a new independent femininity. One might assume that because women were no longer wearing dungarees, burning bras and calling for the end of men, that feminism and feminists had vanished. That would be a very mistaken assumption. As far as the academy and universities in particular were concerned, feminism was just getting going.

Prior to 1990, as I stated in Chapter 2, Marxist theory and its numerous variations dominated sociological theory, research and methodology.[97] From 1990 onwards and the introduction of poststructuralism, including feminist poststructuralism (also postmodernism) the Marxists and Neo-Marxists were on the back foot. They stayed on the back foot throughout the 1990s, eventually conceding to the feminists during the noughties. Nowadays, it is not Marxism that prevails in universities across Europe, Australasia, North America, or even South Asia and East Asia: it is feminism and its variants. The layperson may call it 'identity politics', 'culture wars' or 'woke' but for the intellectual it is 'post-colonial theory', 'psychoanalytical feminism', 'feminist poststructuralism', 'intersectionality', 'critical race theory', 'eco-feminism', 'Chicana feminism' and 'Black feminism'.[98] In short,

---

[96] For an introduction and overview of feminist theories, see Whitehead, Talahite and Moodley, (2013). For an in-depth examination, see Tong and Botts (2024).

[97] A prominent example from that period are the debates (often heated!) within Organisational Behaviour and Organisational Studies, especially between Labour Process Theory/Theorists (largely Marxist, neo-Marxist in orientation), and the postmodernists, poststructuralists and varied feminist theoreticians. https://www.sciencedirect.com/topics/social-sciences/labor-process-theory; https://discourseanalyzer.com/introduction-to-post-structuralism-in-discourse-analysis/

[98] See Tong and Botts (2024) for examples, definitions and comparisons.

in a generation, and driven by intellectuals and researchers in countless numbers of universities, feminism had progressed from being seen as primarily reflecting the concerns of Western white middle-class women to becoming a worldwide movement speaking for and representing women across both the Global North and Global South.

To put the importance of this in context: throughout the 1950s less than 2% of women went to university and most of these were trainee teachers. By 2000, that had risen to over 60% and these female students were studying everything from quantum physics to leadership and management.[99] And this wasn't only in the West: the historic massification of higher education since the 1970s is recognised as a worldwide phenomenon,[100] a hallmark of globalisation, with student enrolments 'accelerating dramatically in every type of country from the 1960s onwards'.[101] This worldwide expansion of higher learning is a defining factor in the social changes now impacting the twenty-first century – and it is women, not men, who have been at the forefront of this transformation both in terms of enrolment numbers and educational achievements. It was at university that many millions of women around the world received their first real exposure to feminism as theory, philosophy and practice, as did large numbers of men.

Some of these women and men will have graduated considering themselves to be feminists. Not all, but some. But all will have graduated considering themselves educated, modern, enlightened, non-traditional and independent-minded.

If we have to thank one body of people for the survival of feminism and the subsequent rise in independent femininity, it is the hitherto unsung heroines and heroes of the academy: the many thousands of lecturers and

---

[99] https://journals.openedition.org/osb/1563?lang=en https://www.russellsage.org/news/rise-women-seven-charts-showing-womens-rapid-gains-educational-achievement; https://dera.ioe.ac.uk/id/eprint/8717/1/DIUS-RR-08-14.pdf https://www.theglobaleconomy.com/rankings/Female_to_male_ratio_students_tertiary_level_educa/ https://www.insidehighered.com/news/2013/02/21/new-book-explains-why-women-outpace-men-education

[100] https://higheredstrategy.com/four-megatrends-in-international-higher-education-massification/

[101] Schofer, E. and Meyer, J.W. (2005) 'The Worldwide Expansion of Higher Education in the Twentieth Century, in *American Sociological Review,* Vol. 70, December, pp. 898-920. Also, https://link.springer.com/article/10.1007/s10734-016-0016-x

professors who – over the decades but especially from the 1980s – nurtured feminism, developed feminist theories (especially concepts such as diversity, equity, inclusion and justice), researched and published books and journal articles grounded in the principles of feminist enquiry and methodology, and taught all this to many millions of students.

Out of this rising mass of educated humanity have emerge adults sensitised to issues and contestations regarding identity, agency, choice, ethics, community and individuality. These are the political and philosophical underpinnings to the new independent femininity now abroad in our societies and communities. Before we look more closely at independent femininity it is necessary to examine just what it has replaced.

Traditional/Hegemonic Femininity – Internalised Patriarchy

Hegemony is a concept originated by Antonio Gramsci, a Marxist philosopher from the early twentieth century. Simply defined, it refers to *'how powerful groups in society use language, education, culture and ideology (such as the media) to make their dominant position look "normal" and "natural" to the larger population.'*[102] In the late 1980s, Raewyn Connell placed hegemony alongside masculinity and produced 'hegemonic masculinity'; i.e. traditional – or in today's everyday parlance, toxic – masculinity.[103]

Since the 1990s, hegemonic masculinity has become the 'go-to' concept for sociologists studying men and masculinities, and I undertook a detailed examination and critique of the concept in my first academic book (2001).[104] However, what has been overlooked in sociology is the possibility of a hegemonic femininity, the reason probably being that applying 'hegemonic 'to femininity seems counterintuitive or possibly an oxymoron: a contradiction in terms i.e. if women have reduced power in a patriarchal system how can they apply hegemony?

Well, women can certainly apply power, and have done for centuries. Unfortunately for women as a global gender group, the power they have expressed has been within a conditional gender system that compromised them by virtue of being named 'the Other' to men; the 51% minority. Within this marginalised state, which in many cultures amounted to

---

[102] Whitehead, Talahite and Moodley (2013). P. 18.

[103] Connell, R.W. (1995) *Masculinities.* Cambridge: Polity.

[104] Whitehead, S.M. (2001) Chapter 3.

gender apartheid (see Chapter 4), women developed a femininity which corresponded to, and indeed emphasised, their reduced status. For millennia the vast majority of women certainly expressed a feminine identity and thereby exercised some power of self-identification; unfortunately it was a 'patriarchal-defined feminine identity association' producing a toxic way of being female: toxic, that is, in terms of acting to reduce women's agency.

> 'Patriarchal-defined feminine gender identity association, or traditional femininity, is the internalization and expression of traditional gender values arising from a patriarchal system. While these values can offer women a sense of positive femininity because they align with the gender order, they can also create feelings of shame, guilt, rejection, frustration, neglect, confusion, disenchantment, abuse, violence, and hopelessness; a state of being wherein the woman presents her self only for the judgement and consumption of men and others, not for her innate well-being.'[105]

My research shows how traditional femininity manifests in a woman's sense of self, thereby providing a discursive framework for being and becoming a feminine subject: woman. However, its primary conditions are silence, passivity, frustration, guilt, shame and collusion. In some women it can trigger self-loathing, depression and related illnesses.

> 'Toxic femininity is the noxious, always dangerous, potentially lethal condition which takes root in a woman when she fails to recognise her true value as a woman, as a human being; and especially when she uncritically adheres to gender rules and regulations requiring she conform to traditional feminine values – mostly to suit men. In other words, when she is not living an authentic life – her life – but is instead striving to meet the unrealistic, unhealthy, gendered and sexually objectified expectations of men.'[106]

[Note that the very opposite condition applies with hegemonic masculinity, in that men gravitate towards and adopt this way of being and becoming a man not in order to fulfil women's expectations of them but other men's expectations of them.]

---

[105] Van, Thanh Binh and Whitehead, S. (2025) *The Myths of Toxic Femininity: Causes, Consequences and Cure.* London: Acorn Books. P.10.

[106] Ibid p. 11.

Traditional femininity has had a hegemonic effect, a dominance or influence over females for centuries and always it has been enforced physically, educationally, religiously and culturally, while being validated and approved by men. To see its contemporary manifestation as gender apartheid, look no further than Afghanistan and Iran in the twenty-first century. In essence, the discourses surrounding traditional femininity attempt to internalise women's adherence to their own subjectification and minority state. And once such a femininity is internalised it is unlikely to be questioned by the female: she becomes that which a patriarchal system – men – requires her to become. In feminist poststructuralist terms, she becomes the discourses available to her.

In short, the whole point of hegemonic femininity is to maintain females/women in a state of ignorance and acceptance as to their marginalised reality, to minimise resistance to male power and abuse, and where possible to ensure women collude and cooperate in those practices that serve to subjugate women and reduce their agency, e.g. when women actively support and ensure the FGM (female genital mutilation) of young girls and women.[107]

While all this may sound horrific for women, which it is, resistance to male power in all its many layers – material, psychological, political and cultural – is not straightforward for women and never has been through history.

To give an example, a female born into the majority working class in Victorian Britain was to be born without property rights, education, political rights, or control over body and sexuality, and to be denied access to positions of authority. She had little or no agency in her life. If she had employment it was likely to be as a servant, millworker, factory-worker or farmworker and without any employment rights.[108] Spinsterhood was not a desirable state: a poor woman could not afford to live alone, financially or for her physical safety. Women needed a male 'protector' otherwise they were extremely vulnerable – and most women were still vulnerable with a 'male protector' as domestic abuse was legitimised in law. Working-class

---

[107] UNICEF estimates over 230 million girls and women alive today have been subjected to female genital mutilation; a 15% increase in the number of FGM survivors compared to data released in 2016. https://www.unicef.org/press-releases/over-230-million-girls-and-women-alive-today-have-been-subjected-female-genital

[108] See, for examples and elaboration, Groom, B. (2022) *Northerners: A History*. Manchester: Harper North.

women especially were condemned to become child-producing machines in a world dominated by men and patriarchal values.[109]

That was the condition of women in Victorian Britain; it was even worse in other parts of the world, a reduced state that remains visible in many countries to this day.

It wasn't easy for a British woman in the Victorian era, or the eras before that, to resist hegemonic femininity and strike out for a totally independent lifestyle. Indeed it was virtually impossible, especially for a woman on her own; the material conditions were against her as were the prevailing gender rules, roles and assumptions. Yet there has always been resistance. Looking back over time we see can how a few women, those not born to power, learned to express their femininity and sexuality, and subsequently exercise power and influence in a world where they remained the 'Other'; invariably doing so through marriage to powerful men and/or seduction of powerful men (e.g. Catherine the Great; Anne of Cleves, Wu Zetian and in the first half of the last century, Eleanor Roosevelt, Pamela Churchill Harriman and Eva Peron).[110]

It is the few examples which prove the rule: traditional femininity, reinforced by compulsory heterosexuality, has had hegemonic dominance over the lives and subjectivities of women down the ages, thereby reducing not just their material opportunities but to a large extent determining their very sense of being. The hegemonic capacity of traditional femininity lies

---

[109] See, for discussion, Perkin, J. (1994) *Victorian Women*. London: John Murray. Also, Booth, A.L. (2024) *Women in Victorian Society*. London: Amberley Publishing.

[110] Catherine the Great: Massie. R.K. (2011) *Catherine the Great. Portrait of a Woman*. London: Head of Zeus.

Anne of Cleves: Norton. E. (2010) *Anne of Cleves: Henry VIII's Discarded Bride*. London: Amberley Publishing.

Wu Zetian: Rockefeller, L.A. (2016) *Empress Wu Zetian. (Legendary Women of World History Book 5)*. New York: L.A.Rockefeller Books.

Eleanor Roosevelt: Gerber, R. (2003) *Leadership the Eleanor Roosevelt Way*. New York: Portfolio.

Pamela Churchill Harriman: Purnell, S. (2024) *Kingmaker: Pamela Churchill Harriman's Astonishing Life of Seduction, Intrigue and Power*. London: Virago.

Eva Peron: Hedges, J. (2016) *Evita: The Life of Eva Peron*. New York: I.B.Tauris.

precisely in the way it is culturally presented as the most desirable and natural way of being female, a discursive condition reinforced via religious and legal sanction, often with the threat of male violence attached. That this way of being a woman happens to correspond with traditional masculinity, thereby fitting neatly into the patriarchal arrangement, invariably gets overlooked, or was until women changed the rules, created an alternative way of being a woman, and set forth on a path which was non-traditional, liberating and agentic.

The gender revolution, noticeable from the 1950s and accelerating into the subsequent decades of the twentieth century, has emerged as the global phenomenon of the twenty-first century. This revolution, at its core, is a rejection of traditional ways of being a woman – hegemonic femininity – together with the limitations and abuses that such a femininity 'justifies' and mythologises as 'natural and biologically inevitable'.

As described in Chapter 2, Simone de Beauvoir was one of the key women who helped open the door to this possibility and indeed predicted it in her writings, though perhaps even she didn't fully appreciate the breadth and depth of the gender revolution, nor how it would come to impact on the lives of women in every country and every culture. If de Beauvoir did at times envisage a new, healthier more liberated way of being a woman, then it would likely have looked something akin to independent femininity.

Defining Independent Femininity

As I have stressed, there have always been women with a feisty attitude, who resisted patriarchy and male abuse, and who demonstrated a strong, independent character. As I described in the previous chapter, my family was full of such women. But notwithstanding their ability to control or at least resist those men around them when they needed to, none of these women could escape internalising the discourses of traditional femininity; these discourses – as languages, beliefs and practices – were just too powerful, too normalised in culture and too entrenched with male and female roles and the gendered public and private spheres that structured society. This resulted in few women rejecting traditional femininity simply because (a) they didn't see their traditional feminine values as a problem for their agency and (b) the patriarchal system severely limited their opportunity to be independent.

And yet here we are, a quarter of the way into the twenty-first century, and already it is plain to anyone who cares to look that women have changed and are doing so with some alacrity. No matter that there is a backlash, mostly from men and examined in the subsequent chapter: that is to be expected. The point is that women have normalised a new and liberating way of being a woman. It is also important to stress that most of the women doing this are straight. They are not all LGBTQ+. And being straight they have a difficult path to tread because their biological sexuality and impulse is towards the male. It is one thing for a lesbian to declare she wants nothing to do with men and can happily live without them; it is rather different if the woman is straight – and most are.

Nevertheless, and as I detail in the final chapter, this is the direction the gender revolution is heading; not towards lesbian feminists rejecting relationships with men – that would not be a revolution but merely be a continuation of biological sexuality – but towards straight women rejecting or limiting their relationships with men. That is the drastic and historic reordering at the core of the gender revolution and that is what will inevitably change society with the potential to bring about 'the end of sex'.

So, in what ways is independent femininity different to traditional femininity? How does a woman with independent femininity express it?

1. Emphasises self-expression, agency and freedom to choose her lifestyle.

2. Will not tolerate abuse, violence and harassment from any male.

3. Able and prepared to articulate her political position and stand by it.

4. Comfortable in her sexuality and able to assert and express it when she feels the need.

5. Does not require, nor seek, a man to act as her protector.

6. If not a declared feminist, will be pro-gender equality (though they amount to the same thing).

7. Does not seek permission from anyone, especially prominent men in her life, to follow her own path.

8. Financially independent, or aims to be.

9. Has high levels of self-awareness and self-appreciation and therefore does not rely on love validation from a man in order to feel complete.

10. Considers men no more than her equal as a gender, not her superiors.

11. Demands to have control over her fertility and reproductive system.

12. Is determined to fashion her sense of self and her identity unrestricted by maleist oversight, sanction and control.

It should be recognised that the independent femininity I am describing comes with certain conditions and provisos. For example, it is much easier for a middle-class educated woman with a professional identity to espouse an independent femininity than it is for a poor, working-class woman with little or no cultural capital.[111] That said, research I have co-conducted shows that there are interventions which can be made into the lives of most any woman whatever her class, race, ethnicity and economic situation, resulting in an increase in her self-confidence, self-appreciation, self-protection, self-management and agency.[112] Additionally, should a woman with independent femininity marry and have children, then that would inevitably impact on some of the above criteria; compromises and accommodations would have to be made, both with partner and with the children. This could be one reason for the 'gender divergence' described in Chapter 5.

It is also important to note that independent femininity does not preclude any lifestyle or political choice, as long as it is made by the woman freely and is therefore not subject to male enforcement. This means that not all women with independent femininity are going to be liberal-minded, woke, and pro-LGBTQ+, nor indeed anti-racist. A large number of such women voted for Donald Trump in the 2024 US Presidential Election, voted for the Conservative Party and Reform UK in the 2024 UK General Election, and frequently vote for various right-wing political parties elsewhere around the world. This may appear a confusing anomaly to many political commentators and gender theorists, but it is entirely predictable. As I have long emphasised, *there are as many if not more differences within the categories of male and female as there are between these two categories*. How people vote in a democratic election does not automatically translate into

---

[111] https://www.oxfordreference.com/display/10.1093/oi/authority.20110803095652799

[112] See, Van Thanh Binh and Whitehead, S. (2024) *Self Love for Women*. Acorn Books. Based on thirteen case studies, this book evidences the importance and power of totally inclusive self-love for enabling women to recognise and discard constraints arising from toxic/hegemonic femininity.

how they see themselves as gendered individuals and nor does it assume such women to be passive 'cultural dopes' of toxic males/masculinity. There are a host of other factors that individuals take into consideration when determining who to vote for, not least employment, economics, physical safety, career, family, personal wellbeing, national security, immigration and national identity.

> *This is how intersectionality comes to influence democratic elections while making the outcomes inherently unpredictable – no one person having only one aspect of their identity to invest in; every identity being a fulcrum around which many differing aspects of the self configure.*

For example, adherence to a religion does not negate the possibility of a woman having an independent femininity. I have met many women of different but persuasive and powerful religions and who follow their religion with dedication; notably Muslim, Catholic, Hindu, Jewish, and Buddhist. While not all are declared feminists (though some are) they most definitely have an independent feminine identity. As one 35-year-old Muslim woman put it to me during a business trip I made to Damascus in 1995:

> *"I married an older professor from my university when I was 28, all approved and supported by family. But after marriage he tried to control my life, dominate me. I couldn't accept it. We were divorced a few years later. My family didn't want me to get divorced but it was my choice. None of this means I am any less of a Muslim. I am strong believer and follower of Islam. The problem is the attitude of so many Muslim men, not the religion itself."*

Just a few examples from within my personal and professional network:

- A British professor and strong feminist who runs a daily Catholic prayer group.
- A Millennial Indian woman, single, professional, strongly independent minded, who is a dedicated Hindu.
- A confident, independent-minded Thai woman, company CEO, who is an avowed Buddhist and follower of certain Thai Buddhist masters.
- A Jewish UK Professor, long-time notable feminist and well-published academic, who closely follows her religion.

- A Vietnamese Millennial woman, university professor, counsellor, divorcee and independent female, disciple of the late Vietnamese monk, Thich Nhat Hanh.
- A Malaysian Christian woman, CEO of several companies, very independent minded and promoter of women's rights and LGTB identities and also very spiritual and religious.
- An Indonesian Muslim woman in her forties, married with children, promotor of women's rights and independence, International School Director, strong Muslim beliefs.
- A Black British woman, lawyer and feminist, who is also a Creationist.

When considering the growing ubiquity of independent femininity we should remain sensitive to differences within the population of women. We must recognise the intersectionality of women's identities, together with their ability to accommodate potentially contradictory if not conflicting identity elements. While I have posited a list of criteria for independent femininity, not all women will express these criteria in exactly the same way nor with the same degree of consistency and commitment. As I explained in Chapter 1, all identity is discursive and intersectional and so is independent femininity, making any attempt to predict individual behaviour highly risky.

This is precisely where feminism and independent femininity part company: the former is a dominant discourse that promotes equality for all, or what I term total inclusivity, and that encourages the individual to be active in promoting DEIJ (Diversity, Equality, Inclusion and Justice). To be feminist is, therefore, to believe in the following:

> 'Total Inclusivity means recognising, valuing, protecting and nurturing diverse identities, including those of race, gender, sexual orientation, class, disability, age, religion and language.'[113]

In contrast, independent femininity has no underpinning ideology or dominant discourse: it is nothing more or less than the internationalised expression of an individual woman's desire for, and intent to have, an independent life. And by independent, I mean independent from men as rulers, controllers, dictators, abusers or protectors – patriarchs. How a woman with independent femininity lives her life is up to her – which is the whole point of it.

---

[113] Whitehead, S. (2022) *Total inclusivity at Work*. London: Routledge. P. 2.

To give an example – one highly pertinent at time of writing – a woman with independent femininity might find herself being able to vote for Donald Trump as President. A feminist most definitely could not.

In terms of quantifying this gender revolution, is it possible to estimate the number of women around the world with independent femininity?

Well, we can assume that all feminists have a desire to live their lives with agency and choice, free from male domination, which, based on recent research, immediately accounts for, say, 35% of women,[114] at least in all high- and upper-income countries. But what about the remaining 65% not declaring as feminist? How many of these women, especially Gen Z and Millennial, are still adhering to traditional femininity at this stage in the twenty-first century? From the trends we are seeing in women openly rejecting traditional gender roles and cultures (see Chapter 5) and publicly expressing anger, frustration and resistance to male dominance, male violence and patriarchal control (including in countries that are not high- and upper-income, such as Afghanistan, Turkey, Iran, South Africa, Mexico, Russia, Pakistan and Peru), then for sure traditional femininity is rapidly being replaced by independent femininity. But even if we estimate only 50% of non-feminist women to have an independent femininity, say 32% in total, and add that to the 35% of feminists, then we are at 67% of all women worldwide, and my guess is that it's somewhat higher than that, especially with Gen Z and Millennial women.

My own unpublished and anecdotal research would suggest the number could be as high as 80% for women under fifty, leaving a diminishing number of older women holding on to traditional femininity. For sure, it is Gen Z and Millennial women around the world who are driving the gender revolution and doing so in increasing number.

And then there are the men supporters, like myself. More on that in the next chapter. But even if there are just 15% of men with what I term a progressive masculinity (and that will be a very conservative estimate), then added to the 65% of women it amounts to billions of us.

To emphasise, the gender revolution is not a feminist revolution: it is a whole lot bigger and more powerful than that. Feminists are certainly part of it, a big part, but this goes further than feminism – the gender revolution is about identity, both women's and as consequence men's, but predominantly independent feminine identity. Possibly 50% of the world's population are actively changing their sense of who they are as gendered and sexual

---

[114] https://www.statista.com/chart/32523/agreement-with-statement-i-define-myself-as-a-feminist/

beings; engaged in a historic reinvention of femininity and, consequently, masculinity. This is what makes the gender revolution so unique in human history and so potentially earth-shattering in its impact.

To get an understanding of the gender revolution's magnitude, don't ask a woman whether or not she is a feminist; ask her if she wants, or indeed expects, to live a life of independence, agency and choice.

Factors in the rise of independent femininity from 1990 to present

Although I am describing a 'gender revolution' in this book, it's important to recognise this is a revolution like no other. For one thing, most people don't realise it is happening, not least the women driving it. One reason may be because it appears more like a gender *evolution* than a gender *revolution*. While it is true that gender identity has evolved over the centuries, both for males and females and across all cultures, this has been a slow and steady process rather than a rapid transformation. And by rapid, I mean a dramatic change occurring over less than a century, as has been the case with the gender revolution. Another reason for people not recognising the revolutionary character of these alterations in femininity is because the younger generation don't see the bigger picture. Most Gen Z or indeed Millennial women probably cannot remember a time before the internet, Facebook, the #MeToo movement, mass higher education, sexual freedoms, nor when women weren't in positions of leadership across politics and business. They were born into this revolution; they didn't instigate it. Three generations of females have been born since this revolution really picked up speed in the 1960s, which is one of the benefits of being my age; you get to see a wider perspective having witnessed the changes first-hand.

In this section I list five key global transformations that, taken together, illustrate the dramatic historic rise in independent femininity over the past 35 years: political power, education, careers, social media and globalisation.

Political Power

> *'If Lehman Brothers had been a bit more Lehman Sisters... we would not have had the degree of tragedy that we had as a result of what happened.'* (Christine Lagarde)

One of the most important changes is the political one – because it brings hard power and influence. No surprise, therefore, that women were denied it through history. Unless you were a female born to power, as a Queen, there was little chance of you acquiring it. Even in the USA in the 1970s, when feminism was making its mark on society, men continued to rule the corridors of power: *'mostly, even for the most privileged and intelligent women, the only political role permitted was as hostesses'*.[115] Barely fifty years later and political power now increasingly rests in the hands of women and while women have yet to make the White House as President, they are at least in the running and getting closer. At time of writing, there are 29 countries with female leaders. Since 1960 and the rise of feminism, over a third of countries of the world have been led by women at some point, the USA remaining more resistant to female power than most developed countries.[116] Some notable women political leaders of the past sixty years include Golda Meir (Israel), Margaret Thatcher (UK), Angela Merkel (Germany), Julia Gillard (Australia), Isabel Peron (Argentina), Carrie Lam (Hong Kong), Mary Robinson (Ireland), Giorgia Meloni (Italy), Benazir Bhutto (Pakistan), Park Geun-Hye (South Korea), Jacinda Ardern (New Zealand), Tsai Ing-wen (Taiwan), Indira Gandhi (India), Giorgia Meloni (Italy), Claudia Sheinbaum (Mexico), Michelle Bachelet (Chile) and at time of writing the youngest serving state leader of any country, 36 year-old Kristrun Frostadottir (Iceland).[117]

Have all these women had an easy climb up the political ladder? Absolutely not. Can all of them be considered feminists? No. Are all these women politicians left-leaning, liberal-minded, inclusive and empathetic individuals? No. Did they all have careers untarnished by controversy, failure and criticism? Of course not, they are in politics. Are they all politicians in order to bring about a gender revolution? Most definitely not.

None of which matters to the gender revolution because the point is that these women rose to a position that men have historically dominated and they held it, often in the face of vicious male resistance, resistance which continues in many forms, both physical and online.[118]

---

[115] Purnell, S. (2024) p. 269.

[116] https://www.britannica.com/topic/Which-countries-have-had-women-leaders

[117] In March 2025, an alumni from Keele University, Netumbo Nandi-Ndaitwah, became Nambia's first female president. Another example of global education contributing to the gender revolution.

[118] A growing aspect of global violence against women politicians is the use of AI generated deepfake porn, threatening women's participation in public life. https://www.inkl.com/news/form-of-violence-across-globe-deepfake-porn-targets-women-politicians

As I have emphasised in this book, male and female are not simply two genders, the two core constituencies of the gender binary – they are political categories, and as such they inevitably carry with them more than a single representation. Every woman in politics, just like every woman who has ever lived, carries with her an intersectional, discursive identity, of which 'female' and/or 'woman' is only a part. But it is a vital part because when a woman politician rises to the top of her career then she is visible first as a woman and second as a politician. This is not the situation for male politicians – or hasn't been through history. Male politicians never get judged on their masculinity – though that is now changing – their gender being largely invisible and unacknowledged. For women politicians, their very presence in politics signals dramatic change. In short, independent femininity is inspired to exist by virtue of those women who wield power in the highly public, masculinist political arena, no matter the other aspects of their intersectional identity.[119]

Education

> 'Teach a man; you educate a man. You teach a woman; you educate a generation.' (anon)

One of the most extraordinary and unforeseen aspects of the rise of women is their educational accomplishments.[120] From the 1950s to the 1990s, of primary concern to feminist scholars undertaking educational research was to challenge the *'continued marginalization, stereotyping, and disenfranchisement of women and girls in schools, colleges and universities, and to ensure this 'was not allowed to continue'.*[121] Researchers highlighted the 'gender gap' in male and female educational attainment and it didn't favour the females.[122] However, by 2000 it was becoming clear that a new 'gender gap' had opened up, one that didn't favour the males.[123] This was

---

[119] Women in Governance is just one of many global organisations actively working to 'close the gender gap' and support women in their career advancement and leadership development. https://womeningovernance.world/

[120] See for discussion, DiPerete, T.A. and Buchmann, C. (2013) *The Rise of Women: The Growing Gender Gap in Education and What it Means for American Schools.* New York: Russel Sage Foundation.

[121] https://www.researchgate.net/publication/345429515_Strategic_Feminist_Research_on_Gender_Equality_and_Schooling_in_Britain_in_the_1990s

particularly noticeable in universities: 'a powerful and influential location for the transformation in one's sense of self'.[124] From the 1960s to the mid-1990s, the ratio of male to female students at first-degree level in the UK rose to 50-50. By 2004 that had changed to 42-58. Both male and female student numbers rose strongly from 1994 to 2023, though the increase in female university acceptances was nearly double that of male acceptances during this period. The year it all changed was 1996. Every year since then, more women than men have been accepted to UK universities; in 2023 it was 68,000 students, or 28% more women than men.[125]

This is not just a UK experience but evidenced globally: the ratio of female to male students in tertiary level education in 2021, based on 108 countries, averaged at 1.21%. Meaning there are 21% more female students than male student on average. In the USA it was 1.32%, the UK, 1.26%, Australia 1.33%, with the highest-level being Qatar at 1.79%.[126]

The Netherlands (1.14%) is typical of many of these countries in having had more women than men in higher education for almost a quarter of a century.[127] That means a global generation of women growing up in a world where not only are they getting into university but they expect to do so.[128] The difference from the 1950s could not be starker.

---

[122] Arnot, M., David. M.E., and Weiner, G. (1999) *Closing the Gender Gap: Postwar Education and Social Change*. Cambridge: Polity.

[123] https://www.brookings.edu/articles/boys-left-behind-education-gender-gaps-across-the-us/ Note that globally, a 'gender gap between rich and poor girls' continues and will 'take a long time to close' https://www.brookings.edu/articles/the-uss-role-in-advancing-gender-equality-globally-through-girls-education/

[124] https://www.universityworldnews.com/post.php?story=20190408084550435

[125] https://www.insidehighered.com/news/2013/02/21/new-book-explains-why-women-outpace-men-education

https://researchbriefings.files.parliament.uk/documents/CBP-7857/CBP-7857.pdf

[126] https://www.theglobaleconomy.com/rankings/Female_to_male_ratio_students_tertiary_level_educa/

[127] https://schengen.news/women-outnumbered-men-in-dutch-universities-for-23rd-consecutive-year/

[128] https://www.cbs.nl/en-gb/news/2023/10/more-women-than-men-in-higher-education-for-23-consecutive-years

However, this aspect of the gender revolution is not just about numbers. Women are now outperforming men in every level of education from kindergarten to PhD,[129] not just in the UK and USA but in most middle- and high-income countries.[130]

The subsequent Impact on women's self-esteem, aspirations, employment opportunities, choice of partners, lifestyle options, income levels and sense of identity cannot be overstated. There are clearly identifiable links between women's educational level and their access to material resources, decision-making abilities and agency.[131]

> 'Girl's education... has often been cited as the world's best investment, the key to enabling girls and women more agency in their homes, communities and countries.'[132]
>
> 'The education and professional careers of women also have a significant influence on the modernization of family relations and the move towards gender equality. Women who are educated and financially independent are better equipped to challenge traditional gender roles and to demand equal treatment in all aspects of their lives.'[133]

I've been an educator since the mid-1980s. Not only has higher education empowered me, changed my life and my identity, but I have also been fortunate and privileged to see close-up how it empowers and changes others; people of all ages, genders, sexes, races, ethnicities and nationalities. No matter the country, no matter the culture, education changes lives for the better and it certainly changes women's lives for the better. No doubt the male-dominated political systems around the world did not decide from the

---

[129] https://spartanshield.org/42176/feature/its-a-girls-world/

[130] https://www.forbes.com/sites/nickmorrison/2024/01/14/from-kindergarten-to-college-girls-are-outperforming-boys/

[131] https://www.linkedin.com/pulse/importance-education-womens-individual-agency-gender-equality-gitahi

[132] Sperling, G.B. and Winthrop, R. (2015) *What Works in Girls' Education. Evidence for the world's best investment.* New York: Brookings Institute Press.

[133] https://www.imf.org/en/News/Articles/2015/09/28/04/53/sp060614

https://www.un.org/en/chronicle/article/education-pathway-towards-gender-equality?t

1960s onwards to empower women and girls through opening up education and creating a massification of higher education, but empowerment is the result of those actions. Without question, the individual empowerment and agentic potential that comes from education is one of the most important factors in pushing forward the gender revolution over the past half-century or more. Is it the most important factor? I don't know. But it seems unlikely that we'd be this far into the global gender revolution without the corresponding global educational revolution.

Careers

> 'Let woman choose her own vocation just as a man does his. Let her go into business, let her make money, let her become independent, if possible, of a man.' Maggie Lena Walker

In just seven decades we've gone from an age when women couldn't wear trousers in public without being criticised, and certainly not in flashy New York restaurants, to where they control large swathes of business and commerce. Notwithstanding that there is much room left for greater representation, plus the fact that women still do not receive equal pay for equal work with the gender pay gap stubbornly enduring,[134] over the past thirty years women have left the home and entered the office if not the boardroom in impressive numbers.

- 42% of all US businesses are owned by women.
- Women-owned businesses have grown by 114% in the last two decades.
- About half of start-ups in the US are founded by women.
- One third of businesses worldwide are owned by women.
- One in four businesses have female owners in low-income countries.
- Globally, in 2022 women occupied 42.7% of all senior and leadership roles.
- Globally, one in five start-ups had at least one woman founder in 2019.[135]

---

[134] https://www.pewresearch.org/short-reads/2023/03/01/gender-pay-gap-facts/

[135] https://luisazhou.com/blog/women-in-business-statistics/

What is also noticeable is the way women have begun assuming top leadership positions in professions and domains hitherto totally dominated by men. Examples in the UK include the police: 50,000 women police officers and 40% of Chief Constables. Fire service: 2017–2019, first woman commissioner of the London Fire Brigade; women firefighters at 8.7%, – 2,985 up from 1,755 in 2013. British Army: 16,220 women in the UK regular forces, comprising 11.7% of total, with the first woman general appointed in 2024. Universities: the percentage of female Vice Chancellors running UK universities has more than doubled in the past twenty years to 24%.[136]

The countries with the most women in political and business leadership are Austria, the UK and Argentina. The country with the highest percentage of women CEOs is Norway (13.4%) followed by Singapore, Thailand, Sweden and Taiwan.[137]

Globally, the employment sectors where women have the highest representation in senior leadership positions are Health and Care Services (49.5%); Education (46.0%); Consumer Services (45.9%), Government and Public Sector (40.3%); Retail (38.5%); Entertainment Providers (37.1%); and Administrative and Support Services (24.7%). The number of women hired into leadership positions is increasing, but slowly.[138] In terms of science, women remain in a minority of researchers at approximately 33.7% across 107 countries, though the number is rising steadily. The regions with the highest percentage of female scientists/researchers in 2021 are Central Asia (49.6%); Latin America and Caribbean (44.4%); and the Arab States (41.4%). In the EU, of the 78.3 million employed in science and technology in 2022, 52% are women, a doubling in less than ten years.[139,140]

---

[136] https://www.telegraph.co.uk/news/2023/01/09/record-40-per-cent-chief-constables-now-women-amid-anti-misogyny/ https://www.theguardian.com/news/2017/mar/12/big-issue-first-female-boss-needs-wit-and-talent-to-restore-fire-service https://commonslibrary.parliament.uk/representation-of-women-in-the-armed-forces/ https://en.wikipedia.org/wiki/Sharon_Nesmith#:~:text=In%20May%202024%2C%20it%20was,female%20officer%20in%20British%20history.

[137] https://www.investmentmonitor.ai/news/countries-women-business-political-leadership-positions/?cf-view

[138] https://economicgraph.linkedin.com/blog/the-number-of-women-hired-into-leadership-is-increasing-but-by-less-than-one-percent-a-year

[139] https://unesdoc.unesco.org/ark:/48223/pf0000388805#:~:text=Looking%20only%20at%20the%20data,2015%20to%202018%20%5Biv%5D. https://

Of course, statistics only tell part of the story. They do not reveal the individual obstacles which countless numbers of women continue to face at work; harassment, discrimination, stereotyping, unequal pay and conditions,[141] the 'boy's own' work culture,[142] bullying and silencing. Yet nor do they account for the relationship an individual has with work beyond the material – the salary. Work has long been acknowledged as playing a vital role in the construction of identity and validation of the self, the ego, and this is especially true for women, historically denied access to careers and self-actualisation through paid employment. Not only are women now in work and developing careers across a range of industries and professions, they are doing so with great success. Indeed, recent studies show that Gen Z women in the UK, for example, are more likely to be in employment than men and are 'out-earning their male peers'.[143] We must certainly fight for improvement while also recognising that the transformation in women's lives, aspirations, opportunity for independent lifestyles since the 1950s, underpinned by widening career possibilities, is unquestionably historic and momentous.

---

ec.europa.eu/eurostat/web/products-eurostat-news/w/ddn-20240613-2#:~:text=Of%20the%2078.3%20million%20people,technology%20employed%20in%20service%20activities. https://www.weforum.org/publications/global-gender-gap-report-2023/in-full/gender-gaps-in-the-workforce/#:~:text=The%20sectors%20where%20gender%20diversity,Retail%20(38.5%25)%2C%20Entertainment%20Providers https://www.investmentmonitor.ai/news/countries-women-business-political-leadership-positions/ https://www.investmentmonitor.ai/news/countries-women-business-political-leadership-positions/

[140] Global women's labour-force participation rate declined between 2019 and 2020 by 3.4% compared to 2.4% for men, it increased to 64% by 2023, accounting for approx. 40% of the global workforce. https://www.weforum.org/publications/global-gender-gap-report-2023/in-full/gender-gaps-in-the-workforce/

[141] https://www.pewresearch.org/short-reads/2023/03/01/gender-pay-gap-facts/

[142] See for example, Kerfoot, D. and Whitehead, S. (1998) "Boy's Own Stuff": masculinity and the management of further education, *The Sociological Review*. 46(3) August. Also, Whitehead, S. (2022) *Total Inclusivity at Work*.

[143] https://www.independent.co.uk/life-style/the-gen-z-gender-pay-gap-has-reversed-so-what-s-up-with-boys-b2761997.html

Social Media

'Disrupt to innovate! We live in wonderful times, where acceptance for change is getting far easier. Don't just talk about breaking the glass ceiling, build your own.' Pooja Trehan.

So far, I have made only minor reference to India and even less to China, yet no convincing elaboration of the gender revolution can be had without noting the importance of these two countries, each with some 690 million females – nearly 1.4 billion females or approximately 28% of the global female population.

The force and diversity of influences on India and China since the 1950s is recognised to be enormous and far beyond the aims and scope of this book. So I will take just a single variable, one which now impacts most every human on earth: social media.

Accepting that social media is not benign and can never be, nor that it has been carefully designed as a liberating, safe, healthy space for humans to interact – cyberbullying, stalking, and trolling of women being commonplace – it is nevertheless a crucial part of the gender revolution, especially for Indian and Chinese women.[144]

India now has the second-largest number of internet users globally (862 million), though only 43% of Indians have internet access. The average user spends 2.6 hours daily on social media platforms and 54% of Indians go to social media channels to find "truthful" information, compared to a global average of 37%. WhatsApp has the largest user base followed by Instagram and Facebook. While more Indian males than females use social media, between 27% and 30% of all females are regular social media users, the highest number being in the 18–34 age-group – 38%.[145]

Despite India being a country with deeply embedded notions of hegemonic masculinity and hegemonic femininity, high levels of male violence against women and domestic abuse, misogyny and institutionalised sexism, all compounded by the many racial, religious and ethnic tensions

---

[144] https://www.academia.edu/20842006/The_Role_of_Social_Media_in_Enlightening_Women_on_Gender_Issues_An_Empirical_Study?email_work_card=title https://www.academia.edu/37984447/Impact_of_Social_Media_on_Indian_Society_towards_Women?email_work_card=title

[145] https://oosga.com/social-media/ind/ https://blog.emb.global/the-behavior-of-social-media-users/

existing across this vast multicultural society, social media has proved to be an enlightening and emancipatory influence on Indian women.[146]

> 'Social media has transformed the lives of millions [of Indian women] and has been instrumental in connecting the lives of many... Gender issues are the talk of town... Our study reveals that the majority of women have benefitted from social media [via] disseminating information and ideas related to several gender-equality themes and empowering women.'[147]

> 'There are [Indian] women on social media platforms who are the catalysts that bring about positive changes... This Women's Day we can't help but celebrate Indian women who use social media to shine a light on serious issues, shatter stereotypes, and create a more equitable world for women.'[148]

An example of how social media helped fuel Indian women's protests against male violence and misogyny occurred in August 2024, following the rape and murder of a young trainee doctor in Kolkata.[149] Far from being the first such incident in a country where a rape occurs every sixteen minutes, the Kolkata outrage was quickly disseminated across social media resulting in hundreds of thousands of women coming out in protest and to 'reclaim the night'.

Not that India doesn't have a 'litany of laws aimed at protecting women':[150] it does – as do most developed and developing countries – but laws themselves don't change men and their masculinity, nor make for a

---

[146] https://www.outlookindia.com/brand-studio/how-indian-women-are-shaping-the-world-through-social-media https://www.tojqi.net/index.php/journal/article/view/2034

[147] https://www.academia.edu/20842006/The_Role_of_Social_Media_in_Enlightening_Women_on_Gender_Issues_An_Empirical_Study

[148] https://www.outlookindia.com/brand-studio/how-indian-women-are-shaping-the-world-through-social-media

[149] https://www.theguardian.com/global-development/article/2024/aug/23/india-is-outraged-at-a-young-doctors-and-we-have-been-here-too-often?CMP=Share_iOSApp_Other

[150] https://blogs.worldbank.org/en/developmenttalk/indian-womens-long-journey-towards-equality-law-and-practice

safer world for women. A 2024 report[151] revealed that 46% of Indian women fear for their safety when at work and commuting. With Indian women increasingly angry, frustrated – if not desperate – to improve their lives and reduce (ideally eradicate) male violence and discrimination against them, social media is proving to be a most useful weapon. Certainly, social media will be an important reason why India is now a country with one of the highest levels of women declaring themselves to be feminists – 57%.[152]

Sexist and misogynistic as it is, India does at least have a working democracy, something Chinese women have never experienced through their long history. Chinese women live in a highly policed, authoritarian, male-dominated country, ruled by men obsessed with maintaining control at any cost, all reinforced by ancient Confucionist familial values which privilege the gender binary, emphasise distinct male and female roles, and demand acquiescence to male authority. In addition, China has one of the most restrictive media environments in the world, with heavy censorship and a government quick to act against any user who posts 'sensitive information', which includes feminist comment.

Yet despite the powerful cultural and physical restrictions placed on Chinese women, they continue to resist, finding information and inspiration from social media and the realisation that women across China share the same concerns, fears, angers, frustrations and desire to break free from patriarchal control.

> 'Lying in bed one night in 2021, Zhang Zirui was swiping through Weibo when she came across a post that gave her pause. The post, by feminist influencer Lin Maomao, argued that women don't owe their family any obedience. In others, she called on women to be selfish, mean, and not care about their partner, their parents, or anyone but themselves... As Zhang recounted; 'was reading her posts every day and reinvigorating myself. For the first time, I knew women could live differently.'[153]

Over one billion users access social media platforms in China (notably WeChat and TikTok). Some 49% of these users are women; they spend more

[151] https://www.deloitte.com/global/en/issues/work/content/women-at-work-global-outlook.html

[152] https://www.ipsos.com/sites/default/files/ct/news/documents/2024-06/International-Womens-day-2024-report.pdf

[153] https://restofworld.org/2023/china-online-feminist-movement/

time on social media than do men and what attracts a lot of women to social media is the opportunity to voice and resist. One of the most influential digital feminist movements in China, developing over recent years, is the #SeeFemaleWorkers campaign, which highlights marginalised female workers in traditionally male-dominated occupations such as soldiers, firefighters, engineers, couriers and drivers. This movement has inspired feminist discussions, activism, awareness and solidarity across China, positively impacting on Chinese women's growing sense of independent femininity. By April 2020, #SeeFemaleWorkers had 520 million readings and 776,000 discussions.[154]

Just as the #MeToo movement exploded across global social media following its launch by sexual assault survivor Tarana Burke in 2006, being further fuelled by the numerous sexual-abuse allegations against Hollywood film-producer Harvey Weinstein in 2017, Chinese feminists have created their own social media feminist platforms. Not only has #MeToo been adopted by Chinese women since 2006, but also the hashtags #BeenRapedNeverReported and #StandByHer.[155]

One characteristic of Chinese women's resistance to patriarchal oppression is the use of sarcasm, often mixed with comedy. In summer 2024, millions of Tencent Chinese viewers[156] streamed a performance by Chinese female comedian, Caicai, in which she delivers an eight-minute routine about menstruation and men's embarrassment about it. The performance includes the description of an embarrassed delivery man 'attempting to hide an order of sanitary pads in a dark grocery bag'.[157]

---

[154] https://www.tandfonline.com/doi/full/10.1080/14680777.2024.2334782#d1e206

[155] file:///Users/stephenwhitehead/Desktop/mendes-et-al-2023-the-evolution-of-metoo-a-comparative-analysis-of-vernacular-practices-over-time-and-across-languages%20(3).pdf   https://www.sciencedirect.com/science/article/pii/S0747563223000754   https://www.digitalrhetoriccollaborative.org/2020/07/13/stand-by-her-chinese-feminist-rhetoric-during-the-covid-19-pandemic/

[156] Tencent is a highly influential Chinese multinational technology conglomerate, best known for its social media platforms, QQ and WeChat, which collectively connect over a billion users globally.

[157] https://www.scmp.com/opinion/china-opinion/article/3279833/why-chinas-women-are-talking-back-never

Many Chinese men are still stung by a social media comment made by female comedian Yang Li, back in 2020, where she asked: "Why are men so mediocre and yet so confident?"

Despite a flood of protests from Chinese men criticising Yang for this comment, one typical reply in support came from a Chinese woman who pointed out; "So many men are upset because Yang Li speaks the truth". As Yang Li also commented; "If you find it offensive, feel free to watch something else".[158]

Intense Chinese Communist Party efforts to shut down feminist comment on social media, have not stopped gender strife and gender divergence growing in China, with increasing numbers of younger Chinese women defying the traditional gender expectations of their families and Chinese society.

How many women in China are declaring themselves as feminist? One survey, undertaken in 2018, indicates 38% in the 16–64 age group, which is in line with the global average.[159] This would amount to nearly 300 million women. And for every declared feminist in China, as elsewhere around the world, there will be at least another woman with independent femininity, thereby making the majority of Chinese women, and certainly Gen Z and Millennial women, resisting traditional gender values. Combining Indian and Chinese feminists in number gives us a total of around 600 million feminists in these two countries alone, plus an unquantifiable number of women of all ages who would declare themselves to have, or aspire to, an independent femininity, which I would conservatively estimate at approximately two-thirds of all Indian and Chinese women.

Social media hasn't created this situation; men have done that. But what social media has done and is doing increasingly, is providing women with a voice, a connection, a communication, a feminist solidarity, a political platform, and the confidence to realise they are not alone in their frustration, fear, anger and desire to resist male power.

Across both India and China, as elsewhere around the world, many hundreds of millions of women are forging a new sense of femininity: independent femininity. And men are not at the centre of it.

---

[158] https://journals.scholarpublishing.org/index.php/ASSRJ/article/view/12436#:~:text=In%202020%2C%20a%20Chinese%20stand,confidence%3F%22%20in%20the%20show.

[159] https://www.statista.com/statistics/818190/china-perceptions-on-defining-themselves-as-feminist/

Globalisation

> *'You have to act as if it were possible to radically transform the world. And you have to do it all the time.'* (Angela Davis)

All the above influences – political power, education, careers, social media – have one unifying energy source: globalisation. Indeed, it would be fair to say that the rise of globalisation since the 1950s and the corresponding rise of feminism and independent femininity are strongly connected, if not in many ways reinforcing.

Globalisation – 'the increasing interconnectedness of the world as a complex system'[160] – is easy to take for granted seven decades into it, even while it is anything but easy trying to understand all its factors, influences and possibilities. And one of the reasons for this is globalisation's complexity and contradictory character. Globalisation unifies and disperses, controls and disintegrates, brings hope and despair, creates a fortune for some and poverty for others. And so it is with independent femininity. As discussed above, several key empowering, liberalising and enlightening influences have impacted on the lives and subjectivities of countless millions of women around the world over the past 75 years, but at the same time (and I detail it in the following chapter) those same influences have also rendered women and men apart and that divergence is, I argue, accelerating. Human society is at this point of gender divergence, with men in one camp and women in the other, largely because globalisation – and all it has brought with it – has served to expose gendered hegemonic conditions historically entrenched in global society. Globalisation hasn't created this situation; it has only served to expose it. And like any knowledge, once exposed and understood it cannot be unthought, dismissed or rejected.

How many women would not be declared feminists today if it weren't for Harvey Weinstein, #MeToo and Hollywood? Too many to know, though one can now recognise 2006–2017 to be a pivotal decade in the global rise of independent femininity, even if at the time most of us were too busy being appalled at the actions of some famous men than we were in sensing the dramatic and permanent shift in the thinking, attitude and political awareness of women.[161] A decade later and Hollywood, in a signally visible

---

[160] Turner, B.S. and Khondker, H.H. (2010) *Globalization: East and West*. London: Sage.

[161] Mendes, K. , Hollingshead, W., Nau, C., Zhang, J., and Quan-Haase, A. (2023) 'The Evolution of #MeToo: A Comparative Analysis of Vernacular Practices

act of repenting for its many sins against women – or was it simply a skilled marketing attempt to capitalise on a new gender reality? – released the film *Barbie*, described by some academics as 'a landmark film and a way of measuring feminism's place in popular discourse'.[162]

Though to be fair, *Barbie* got to the gender zeitgeist a little late in the day. By the mid-noughties, film and media around the world had already spotted the trend; strong, confident women with independent femininity, 'supported' by weak confused men, many exhibiting the worst conditions of toxic masculinity. These duos have become the mainstay of the media everywhere, typically showing up in films featuring detective/police, the armed forces, law/lawyer or even 'Masters of the Universe' films, not just in Hollywood but also Bollywood, indeed pretty much any place TV series and movies are in production.[163]

Over Time and Across Languages', in *Social Media + Society*, July-September 2023, P. 1-12.

[162] https://www.tandfonline.com/doi/full/10.1080/14680777.2024.2381254

[163] A few notable examples: Prime Suspect; The Fall; Happy Valley; Marcella, Spiral, Loch Ness, Dahaad, Delhi Crime, The Killing, The Bridge, High Country, Mare of Easttown, Criminal Record. Key Characteristics: Female leads are typically portrayed as highly competent, intuitive, and determined. Male characters are often shown struggling with personal issues or professional inadequacies. The women frequently face and overcome institutional sexism and scepticism from male colleagues. These series challenge traditional gender roles in detective fiction, showcasing strong, multifaceted female leads who drive the investigations and story lines.

Other examples of series portraying strong female leads while challenging gender stereotypes; The Queen's Gambit, Killing Eve, Fleabag, It's Okay to Not Be Okay, Kin, I May Destroy You, Yellowjackets, Sweet/Vicious, The Handmaid's Tale, Mrs America, The Glory, Orange is the New Black, Alias, and Revenge.

TV series exploring the concept of toxic masculinity in recent years: Euphoria, You, 13 Reasons Why, Alpha Males, Married at First Sight. Contemporary Western films exploring male sexuality, toxic masculinity and challenging long-held gender stereotypes: The Power of the Dog, Brokeback Mountain, Damsel, The Homesman.

https://www.hola.com/us/entertainment/20240819713422/camila-mendes-masters-of-the-universe-movie/

It is salutary just to reflect on what has taken place amidst us all in just a few short decades.

If you are a Gen Z woman born in, say, 2000 and now aged twenty-four, unless you read your feminist history books you could be forgiven for thinking Harvey Weinstein and his like only arrived on our planet a few years ago.

That would be the totally wrong assumption to make.

Here are just a very few of the many well-known British and American men caught up in accusations (in some instances prosecuted and found guilty) of sexually predatory behaviour since 1940:[164]

---

[164] *Joe Kennedy*: See Purnell, S. (2024)

Louis B. Mayer: See https://en.wikipedia.org/wiki/Louis_B._Mayer

Louis Mountbatten: See Lownie, A. (2019) The Mountbattens: Their Lives and Loves. London: Blink Publishing.

Jimmy Saville: See Davies, D. (2016) In Plain Sight: The Life and Lies of Jimmy Saville

Gary Glitter: See https://www.theguardian.com/news/2024/feb/07/former-pop-star-gary-glitter-must-stay-in-prison-parole-panel-decides

Jonathan King: See https://en.wikipedia.org/wiki/Jonathan_King

Bill Crosby: See https://www.bbc.com/news/topics/c93k0wlpyddt

Roman Polanksi: See https://en.wikipedia.org/wiki/Roman_Polanski_sexual_abuse_case

Cyril Smith: See https://www.bbc.com/news/uk-england-manchester-41655595

Donald Trump: See https://19thnews.org/2023/10/donald-trump-associates-sexual-misconduct-allegations/

Jeffrey Epstein: See https://19thnews.org/2023/10/donald-trump-associates-sexual-misconduct-allegations/

Keith O'Brien: See https://www.theguardian.com/world/2021/sep/05/cardinal-keith-obrien-was-like-god-to-me-then-he-tried-to-seduce-me-the-whistleblowers-tale

Russell Brand: See https://www.latimes.com/entertainment-arts/movies/story/2024-04-29/russell-brand-baptized-christianity-rape-sexual-assault-allegations

Rolf Harris: See https://www.bbc.com/news/uk-60393842

- Joe Kennedy
- Louis B. Mayer
- Louis Mountbatten
- Jimmy Savile
- Gary Glitter
- Jonathan King
- Bill Crosby
- Roman Polanski
- Cyril Smith
- Donald Trump
- Jeffrey Epstein
- Keith O'Brien
- Russell Brand
- Rolf Harris
- Matt Gaetz
- Gerard Depardieu
- Andrew Windsor
- John Smyth
- Mohamed Al Fayed
- Woody Allen

That's just twenty, and the list can go on a lot, lot longer than that. Though these names are enough to prove that Weinstein was not the first only that he was the first to find himself, very unwittingly, as the cause celebre for women (and children) everywhere who are seeking justice, freedom and safety from men.

Matt Gaetz: See https://www.bbc.com/news/articles/cew2z48rp70o

Gerard Depardieu: See *https://www.bbc.com/news/articles/cg5v7ny40q2o*

Andrew Windsor: See https://www.theguardian.com/uk-news/2024/dec/13/from-prince-to-pariah-andrews-never-ending-fall-from-grace

John Smyth: See https://www.theguardian.com/world/2024/nov/16/john-smyth-abuse-report-triggers-existential-crisis-in-church-of-england

Mohamed Al Fayed: See https://www.theguardian.com/world/2024/nov/27/mohamed-al-fayed-may-have-raped-and-abused-more-than-111-women-say-police

Woody Allen: See https://www.nytimes.com/2021/02/05/movies/woody-allen-farrow-accusations.html

A fundamental element in globalised independent femininity is the courage and confidence it offers women to speak out against the violences and harassments they suffer from men. This sense of not being isolated, which many vulnerable women feel, is mediated by the knowledge that there are many others out there with precisely the same fears, experiences and hopes for justice. There are now tens of thousands of individuals and global organisations, including NGOs, monitoring male violence in all its forms in most countries. In the following chapter, I list some of these individuals and agencies – those 'keeping count' of the female victims.

This is the 'information society' in full flow, an elementary part of globalisation.[165] Also in full flow is post-industrialisation, itself central to the information society and now heading fast into its Artificial Intelligence phase.[166] It is worth recalling what the feminist theorists of the 1950s first noticed was the rise of the post-industrial society – the replacement of the traditional manufactory sector with the services sector – and the concomitant change in gender roles; women heading out to work and financial independence. So much that has happened in homes, communities and global society is a direct consequence of post-industrialisation, the rise of advanced technology and the end of male-dominated work. All unforeseen, all unplanned and all unprepared for.

This, fittingly, brings us finally to the 'Butterfly Effect'; a computer model designed by Edward Lorenz in the 1960s which suggested that 'the flap of a butterfly's wings [in the Amazon jungle] might ultimately cause a tornado [in Iowa]'.[167] I'm not sure anyone has applied the 'Butterfly Effect' to feminism and certainly not to independent femininity, but maybe they should. A few (very powerful) 'butterfly effects' on women's consciousness, femininity and subjectivity over the past few decades and worth some scrutiny would, for me, include the Spice Girls, Blackpink, Madonna, Taylor Swift, Jane Fonda, Monica Lewinsky, Lady Gaga, Malala Yousafzai, Princess Diana, Oprah Winfrey, Hillary Clinton, Greta Thunberg, Linda Lovelace, Ruth Bader Ginsburg, Rosa Parks, Alexandria Ocasio-Cortez, Michelle Obama, Indra Nooyi, Melinda Gates, Joanna Lumley, Emma Gonzalez, Linda Cruse and Sheryl Sandberg.

---

[165] https://www.sciencedirect.com/topics/social-sciences/information-society

[166] See, for discussion, Kissinger, H. Schmidt, E. and Huttenlocher, D. (2021) *The Age of AI*. London: John Murray.

[167] https://www.technologyreview.com/2011/02/22/196987/when-the-butterfly-effect-took-flight/

Summary

In the above section on 'education' I asked the question; 'Is education the single most important factor in the rise of women and the subsequent gender revolution?' While I might be personally tempted to answer 'yes', the truth is 'I don't know'. The reality of the gender revolution is far too complex to suggest a single overarching factor or influence because all the factors impact on each other: education does not stand alone – it is not separate from politics, social media, technology, careers, globalisation or even Hollywood and Bollywood movies. These all connect and they all count. And then there are the feminists themselves, the millions of dedicated activists working for decades to bring about change not just in universities and education but every walk of life, from multi-national corporations to religions, from the uniformed services to politics, from unions to the media. Each one of these feminists has played a part, has contributed, and will continue to do so. Indeed, their numbers are likely to swell as the consequences of the gender revolution become more pronounced and more divergent.

This is why the gender revolution cannot be stopped, any more than can be silenced women's growing call and demand for independence, agency, choice, freedom from violence and the opportunity to design their selves not according to traditional gender values and roles, in short to suit men, but according to their own wishes, desires and aspirations.

Independent femininity has been given birth and life by these combined influences and forces and it has all happened with remarkable and historic speed – just seven decades. There is a part of me which looks at this revolution and does see evolution, though perhaps it is too early to claim an evolutionary inevitability to what is now happening to human society. Who knows where it might lead in the great long turn of history? Though the trends are becoming more apparent and more visible, complex as they are. But whenever I find myself confronted by yet another conundrum, contradiction or confirmation of this gender revolution, I see also a single certainty: that once people know something or experience something, it then cannot be unknown nor easily forgotten. And independent femininity is, in the final reckoning, an experience that every woman – no matter her identity – is going to want, indeed is eventually going to demand, and once achieved she will never let it be taken from her. Though as I examine in the next chapter, there are a great many men who now want her back in the patriarchal box. This is not yet a woman-friendly world.

Chapter 4: Men's Responses

"Men are afraid that women will laugh at them. Women are afraid that men will kill them."

Margaret Atwood

The story this book reveals is not a comforting one for men and I know some women have sympathy for their predicament. There they were, busying themselves with the usual stuff that men busy themselves with – war, politics, power, conquest, acquisition, competition, domination, control, sex, reproduction, adventure, building and destroying – forging a world of which they were the undisputed masters, when all the while this masculine monolith was beginning to crumble around them. They never noticed. But then, why would they? After all, men had been the dominant unchallenged species for thousands of years. They lived history, created history and then wrote the history confirming their achievements. The rest – women, the environment, every other species – was expendable, or at best a useful adjunct in men's endless and relentless need to prove themselves, to achieve affirmation of their masculine prowess. Was this not the drive at the heart of every empire ever built – male ego, masculine validation and men's assumption of superiority, with each successive realm together with its inevitable demise, being empirical evidence of what man can 'achieve'?

Twenty-five years into the twenty-first century, and the assumed entitlement that has long accompanied maleness is diminishing before men's eyes. For many men it must feel like being in the legendary Alamo, under siege, hunkered down in their manly fortress peering anxiously at the armies gathered around them: the feminists, the gays, the lesbians, the trans, the queers, the non-binary, those with 'strange pronouns', not forgetting at least a billion independent-minded women – all lumped together as 'woke'. Identifying the enemy as 'woke' serves to distinguish them from the good ol' boys; the hyper-heterosexual tough guys cheering each other up in the last chance saloon, only with Crockett and Bowie now replaced by the likes of Donald Trump, Elon Musk, Xi Jinping, Vladimir Putin and all their wannabes – men stroking their weapons with a familiar fondness, itching to use them. Unfortunately, the 'enemy' gathered around them is not General Santa Anna's army but their daughters, partners, sons, wives, girlfriends, mothers, sisters and brothers; society. Little wonder they feel confused and threatened.

Does all this sound too dramatic, overstated or hyperbolic? Are men really so alarmed by the changes happening around them, by the consequences of the gender revolution? Oh, yes, most definitely. Not all men, but enough. Here is one man's view of the world he's now living in:

> 'The male feminist is the kapo in the concentration camp of the gender wars – they will gas him last. Powerless and castrated, he will dutifully serve their bidding until his death.'[168]

Around the same time as I received the above posting, I received this personal observation on men from a Gen Z Australian cisgender woman:

> 'It's subtle really, the way girls are told to be cautious around boys. We are told if they're mean, it means they like us. So we laugh it off and brush it aside. But it doesn't stop there. Eventually we take the longer route home, hold our keys a little tighter or make phone calls just to feel safer. It just becomes second nature, like an unspoken rule we've learned to follow without question.'[169]

Who is living in the real world, the man in fear of the gender wars and how women will 'disempower and castrate' him before gassing him in a concentration camp, or the young woman reflecting on how she's had to learn to be careful around men, to learn the 'unspoken rules' of survival and safety, *which means learning not to trust men totally?*

Nothing better illustrates the stark and unbridgeable gap between the two genders than the above statements.

And yet all the evidence supports the Australian Gen Z woman, not the frantic, terrorised man, lost in his own maleist nightmare.

At time of writing, France is currently coming to terms with its own evidence that men cannot be wholly trusted, with the trial of 51 of them accused of the rape or sexually assault of 72-year-old Gisele Pelicot, aided and abetted by her then husband Dominique, also aged 72. Apparently, her

---

[168] Comment received on 23rd October, 2024, in response to my answer to the following question: 'Why don't feminists support marginalised men?' https://www.quora.com/profile/Stephen-Whitehead-16

[169] Maddie Graham, 25th October 2024, unpublished essay titled 'My thoughts on modern men'. Personal email communication.

husband liked to give guys (over eighty of them) a 'good time with his wife' first ensuring she was knocked out through a cocktail of drugs. He even filmed the proceedings. This was not a one-off event; it happened regularly over a nine-year period, only ending in 2020. What sort of man would invite eighty men into his home to rape and assault his comatose wife? And what sort of man would accept the invite?

The answer is: any man. OK, not every man for sure, but too many to make rape an exceptional act.

These 51 Frenchmen subsequently convicted for the rape and assault of Gisele are certainly monsters but they are far from being freaks. These are very ordinary men, aged 26 to 74, with occupations as diverse as lorry driver, nurse, journalist, prison warden, soldier and farm worker. Several have previous convictions for assault on women but most have no criminal record. Some are single, some married with children. Yes, everyman.[170]

Who is to blame for this appalling situation, apart that is, from the men standing accused? This is a question France is now agonising over.

The answer lies in a statement made by one of the men:

> 'As the husband had given me permission, in my mind she agreed to it'[171]

A clearer statement of patriarchy in action one couldn't devise. The rapist didn't see himself as a rapist nor committing a violent act against a woman, because her husband 'permitted it'. No agency or choice for Gisele, no compassion for her either. To these men she was just a body, owned by her husband and therefore available to do with as they pleased. She had no identity, no feelings, no agency, no individuality, and they had no guilt, shame or remorse. Well, they may have now but only because they face years in prison.

As Gisele herself put it during the trial: *"It is high time that France's macho, patriarchal society which trivialises rape, changes"*.[172]

We all live together on this planet but in our heads and experiences we inhabit very different worlds and as the mass rape of Gisele Pelicot confirms, the worlds of men and women are very different and increasingly so, with one half apparently still under the impression that the other half is their

---

[170] https://www.theguardian.com/world/2024/dec/19/who-are-the-men-convicted-over-rape-and-assault-of-gisele-pelicot-

[171] Ibid

[172] https://www.bbc.com/news/articles/c1lg2593l8lo

property to do with as they please. If Marilyn French and Andrea Dworkin were alive today they'd simply say to me; "*Stephen, we told you so, all you men are rapists and that's all you are*".

But as a man I know that isn't true. Just as I know that the man who fears that women will put him in a concentration camp is not my ally nor an ally of any woman striking out for independence and safety from men. Whatever world he and men like him inhabit, it's certainly not my world. He's not a pro-feminist, so what is he exactly? Where can we locate him on the spectrum of masculinities? Into which category of men's responses to the rise of feminism and independent femininity do we place this man and those like him? And how many categories are there?

These are really important questions to answer because not all men are the same; not all men are misogynists. Not all men are rapists and abusers. It is just that so many of us are.

Wake Up

Men as a gender group didn't start to wake up to the gender identity changes happening around them and to them until the 1970s, the radical feminist decade during which women confronted men with a very different reality to the one they imagined they were living in. It was like a slow, hesitant awakening from a long, deep sleep. Not all men woke up at once – just a few, but at least it was a start.

One of the first to wake up in the UK was Andrew Tolson. In 1977 he had published a short (146 pages) but powerfully persuasive and impactful book titled *The Limits of Masculinity*, in which he reflectively posed questions related to the 'masculine problem'. Tolson was one of the first men to begin the examination of different types of masculinity; 'middle-class masculinity', 'gay masculinity', 'working-class masculinity', together with the endless dilemmas facing any male desiring a 'masculine identity'.[173]

Not that Tolson had gotten there by himself; as he acknowledged, he was merely following the clues laid down by a growing number of feminist writers from de Beauvoir, Hacker and Hartley in the 1950s to such as Sheila Rowbottom (1973); Ann Oakley (1972) and Eli Zaretsky (1975) in the 70s.[174] By the mid-70s, explicitly pro-feminist 'consciousness-raising' men's groups had emerged in the UK along with a 'British Men Against

---

[173] Tolson, A. (1977) *The Limits of Masculinity*. London: Tavistock Publications.

[174] See, for example, Rowbottom, S. (1973) *Hidden From History*. London: Pluto Press.

Sexism' 'movement.' Though it was all still very much work in progress. As Tolson noted, 'the literature on masculinity itself tends to be haphazard and difficult to find.'[175]

Fifty years ago, it was indeed all rather tentative and piecemeal as far as men critically looking at men and at themselves, was concerned. John Stuart Mill had written *On Liberty and the Subjection of Women*, but that was in the 1850s.[176] Then in the 1970s, American sociologist Joseph Pleck got things moving across the Atlantic with his ground-breaking research into '*The Myth of Masculinity*' and 'the gender sex role paradigm',[177] though it was to take another decade before the critical study of men and masculinities really took off and went global, driven by male pro-feminist sociologists such as Jeff Hearn, R.W. Connell, Michael Kimmel, Arthur Brittan, Peter Nardi and David Morgan.[178] Before the end of this decade, the growth in the number of 'men in feminism' was such that it merited a book of the same title.[179] Not that all feminists were happy about this. I vividly recall a seminar at Leeds Metropolitan University in 1992, presented by a visiting prominent American radical feminist. When I asked her about men researching gender, she slapped me down saying, "we feminists don't need men researching gender". I took the slap but ignored her. Because by then I knew two things about feminists and feminism: (a) There were a good many differences within the feminist movement and many feminists

---

Oakley, A. ((1972) *Sex, Gender and Society*. Melbourne: Temple Smith.

Zaretsky, E. (1976) *Capitalism, Family and Personal Life*. London: Pluto Press.

[175] Tolson, A. p. 151.

[176] Mill, J.S. (1996) [1859] *On Liberty and the Subjection of Women*. Ware: Wordsworth.

[177] Pleck, J.H. (1981) *The Myth of Masculinity*. Cambridge, Mass.: MIT Press.

Pleck J.H. and Sawyer, J. (eds) *Men and Masculinity*. Englewood Cliffs,l NJ: Prentice-Hall.

[178] For examples, see Whitehead, S.M. and Barrett, F.J. (2001) *The Masculinities Reader*. Cambridge, Polity. Also, Whitehead, S.M. (2002) *Men and Masculinities*. Cambridge, Polity. Whitehead, S.M. (2006) *Men and Masculinities: Critical Concepts in Sociology. (Volumes 1-5)*. London: Routledge.

[179] Jardine, A. and Smith, P. (eds) *Men in Feminism*. New York: Routledge.

would not have agreed with her and (b) feminism wasn't going to get very far unless it included men.

Though I also knew the radical feminist had a point, which was that the last thing feminists needed was men colonising feminism. And who could blame her for being wary about that? After all, this was a species quite well known for its colonising instincts.

Shortly after that seminar, and having graduated from my MA, I took the ultimate plunge and headed for a PhD, titled *Public and Private Men: Masculinities at Work in Education Management*. By the time I graduated from my doctorate, in December 1996, I felt a fully paid-up member of the pro-feminist men's movement, a loyalty of association which sustains me to this day, nearly four decades later.

Men Not Understanding Who They Are

If all this sounds rather smooth-going, with men's gender self-awareness increasing by the day, it wasn't. To put this period in context, when I was undertaking my doctoral qualitative research into the gendered subjectivities of male senior leaders in UK Further Education Colleges (1993–1995), I never once mentioned the word, 'masculinity' to those men I was interviewing. I knew if I did that they'd close down immediately. No man back then would have permitted another man to closely question him about his masculinity, and certainly not for a publishable PhD. Masculinity was invisible, forbidden, a no-go area, a confusing, misunderstood, sensitive and dangerous term for men; a highly personal concept few men would have been comfortable discussing or been able to discuss freely. I fully understood that most men would be more comfortable discussing their sex lives with me rather than their masculinity.

Which is why one of my two PhD supervisors, Prof Jeff Hearn,[180] insightfully advised me to ask each of the men I interviewed the following question:

> 'Do you think your experiences in education, as a manager, have in any way been affected by you being a man?'

---

[180] Professor Jeff Hearn (Manchester University) and Professor Sheila Scraton (LMU) were my joint supervisors on my PhD. Jeff being the specialist in the critical study of men and masculinities, Sheila being the lead supervisor and specialist in feminist theory and education. My PhD examiners were Professor Margaret Talbot (internal – LMU) and Professor David Morgan (external – Manchester University).

As I subsequently wrote in my doctoral thesis:

> *'The question seemed to floor these men. On occasions it was as if I had spoken in a foreign language! The majority had no comprehension whatsoever of the question. They appeared never to have reflected on themselves as men; never felt the need to reflect on themselves as men. It was a given: their manhood, masculinity, maleness, were central – a universal 'fact'. It was as if everything else revolved around this. It was like questioning the existence of the sun, sky, or air we breathe:*
>
> Mark: *Mmm… interesting; can you expand on that to help me?*
>
> Kevin: *I don't know… I really don't know how I could answer that.*
>
> Keith: *I don't know… I've just been lucky really.*
>
> Simon: *That is difficult. Difficult to give you a realistic answer… I'm not a woman.*
>
> Rob: *Mmm… [pause]… mmm… another question to ask my wife!*
>
> Jim: *I don't know: I can't answer that.*
>
> Frank: *Don't know: most of my appointments have been women.*
>
> Bill: *No idea… I can't answer that question.*
>
> Howard: *I've never thought about it; I don't treat women differently.*
>
> Merv: *I'm not aware of it, not conscious of it… a difficult question.*
>
> Lawrence: *I don't think so… you can't know.*
>
> Hugh: *Oh God! I don't know… I've always tried to treat men and women similarly.*
>
> Peter: *No, I'm lucky, I've always worked with men.*
>
> Jack: *Difficult to answer that; I've never been a woman.*
>
> *Some made a brave attempt at responding to the question in a positive, reflective way but tended to get lost as they talked, often bringing into their answer points related to 'not knowing women',*

> 'treating them all equally', and so on. Many tended to tail off as they tried to engage with the 'intricacies' of the question:
>
> Nev: Yes, but I'm not sure where I go with that.
>
> Ken: Yes, but...
>
> Greg: I'm not sure; it must have been... yes, it's made a difference.
>
> Gordon: Yes, I tend to be more logical, a systems man.
>
> Len: Yes, because I work in a male-orientated environment.
>
> Len was the only manager who equated the gendered environment in which he lived with his own gender. For all the other managers, any connection escaped them. Certainly, any critical understanding of themselves as 'men' was beyond them. For many, the question was pointless, implying that I should ask women what it meant for them to be men.'[181]

During the research I put the same question to women leaders of Further Education colleges and perhaps not surprisingly got a totally different response. Without exception, the women managers were only too well aware of how being a woman had affected their experiences as education leaders. Indeed, I came to learn that once I asked this question of any woman, it would inevitably cause her to reflect deeply and offer nuanced and enlightening accounts of the relationship between herself as a gender subject, living as a woman, and the male-dominated work environment, indeed society, that she inhabited.

The men I interviewed did not know who they were as men nor how they had come to be that man.

The women knew only too well who they were as women and how they'd come to be that woman.

Moreover, and here is a very important point, my research showed that *women generally know men better than men know themselves; men as a gender group lack the emotional intelligence, self-awareness, self-knowledge and self-appreciation that most women possess.*

---

[181] Whitehead. S.M. (1996) *Public and Private Men: Masculinities at Work in Education Management*. PhD thesis. Leeds Metropolitan University, Leeds, UK. pp.194-195. See also, Whitehead, s. (2001) 'Man': The Invisible Gendered Subject?, in S.M. Whitehead and F.J. Barrett (eds) (2001) *The Masculinities Reader*. Cambridge: Polity.

Therein lies one of the origins of the gender divergence, the separation of the sexes into two polarised camps: self-knowledge. This divergence, fundamental to the historic state of men and exposed by the rise of independent femininity, is not confined to misogynists vs feminists. The much more important and profound division is between self-ignorant men and self-knowing women.

Admittedly, that doctoral study was undertaken over thirty years ago. Maybe the state of men has improved since then; become wiser, developed more emotional self-awareness; with men finally becoming self-knowing as a gender? You can test the veracity of that hypothesis by putting my doctoral question to any man you know and noting the answer.

One thing for sure, thirty years ago there was a deafening silence around men and masculinities. Today, there is not only a whole lot of noise but a whole lot of frustration, anger, disappointment and, perhaps, some possibility. Men have gone from being the 'invisible gendered subject' to being the male subject waiting for the psychoanalyst to declare her verdict on their mental health, which for a lot of men has turned out to be rather worrying.

The Political Responses

In so far as women's power and potential are concerned, men may have been half-asleep for most of their existence, but by the 1990s they were definitely waking up, especially in the USA. One pro-feminist sociologist, Ken Clatterbaugh,[182] identified six major political responses by men to the rise of feminism:

1. *The Conservative Response:* Strongly anti-feminist, drawing on both biological and 'moral' standpoints to argue that traditional gender roles are sacrosanct and should not be challenged.

2. *Men's Rights Response:* Mostly anti-feminist but argues that the focus must now be on the rights of men. Advocates seek to bring legislative changes of benefit to men, especially concerning child custody and divorce.

3. *The Spiritual Response:* Moderately anti-feminist. Exemplified by the writings of Robert Bly and his book *Iron John*.[183]

---

[182] Clatterbaugh, K. (1990) *Contemporary Perspectives on Masculinity: Men, Women and Politics in Modern Society.* Boulder, Col.: Westview Press.

[183] Bly, R. *Iron John.* New York: Addison-Wesley.

Followers believe that feminism and the women's movement are emasculating men from their 'inner selves' and that men need to find their 'archetypal manliness'.

4. *The Socialist Feminist Response:* Aligns with some aspects of feminism, notably social and Marxist feminism. Supporters call for an anti-sexist society but also an anti-capitalist one.

5. *The Group-Specific Response:* Generally pro-feminist but formed around a loose coalition of various racial, religious and ethnic perspectives; e.g. black men, gay men, Jewish men, Latino/Chicano men.

6. *The Pro-feminist Response:* The group most closely aligned to feminism and feminist action; 'pro-feminists are men who seek to develop a 'critique of men's practice' informed by feminism'.[184]

During this period, another American pro-feminist sociologist, Michael Messner,[185] researched the growing number of anti-feminist men's movements, or 'essentialist retreats'; the three primary ones being the Men's Rights Group, the Mythopoetic Men's Movement (MMM) and the Christian Promise Keepers (CPK). Though differing in their objectives, these organisations resisted what their members perceived to be a threat to 'traditional moral values', the 'sanctity of patriarchal marriage', men's 'paternity and divorce rights', and men's 'Zeus power' – e.g. feminists and feminisms.[186]

Some 35 years later all three groups are still around, though having gone through some metamorphosis. The Men's Rights Group has become an elementary part of what is currently commonly referred to as the 'manosphere' (see below) while the MMM is not so much a movement

---

[184] Hearn, J. (1987) *The Gender of Oppression: Men, Masculinity and the Critique of Marxism.* Brighton: Wheatsheaf.

[185] Messner, M. (1997) *Politics of Masculinities: Men in Movements.* Thousand Oaks, Calif.: Sage.

[186] In January 2025, Mark Zuckerberg commented that 'corporate culture needs more masculine energy and less focus on diversity'. This comment has its origins in the myth of male 'Zeus power' and is explicitly anti-feminist, revealing Zuckerberg's adoption, at least in part, of Donald Trump's male fundamentalism. https://www.lemonde.fr/en/economy/article/2025/01/12/mark-zuckerberg-wants-more-masculine-energy-and-less-diversity-policy_6736961_19.html

anymore as a philosophy designed to help men find 'their inner hero' and 'male pride', typically through men's retreats in the US, UK and Australia.

> 'It is December 2018 and a UK company called 'Rebel Wisdom' has organised a retreat for men in a converted workshop in rural Buckinghamshire. The two-day event, called 'The New Masculinity', involves 'metaphorically, going into a cave and confronting the [male] monster inside, eventually returning home with the "treasure" – a more fully integrated personality'.[187]

Of these three groups, the Christian Promise Keepers is the most avidly anti-feminist and altogether less amenable to men subjecting themselves to self-analysis in search of psychological balance and a 'healthier, more self-aware, masculinity'; its members champion chastity, marital fidelity and homophobia, naturally opposing same-sex marriage.

> 'The CPK seeks to promote patriarchal values and relationships; it signals opposition to women exerting choice over reproduction, especially abortion; … it argues that public and private roles are necessarily gendered; and it questions the place of the single parent (mother) in a 'functioning', 'stable' society.'[188]

The CPK eventually assimilated into America's far-right Christian fundamentalist coalition, which now also attracts men from a range of orthodox religions. Members of the Christian right may worship slightly different gods, but they are united in being anti-LGBTQ+, anti-women's rights, anti-feminist, anti-abortion, and largely but not wholly, white supremacist. In the past decade they appear to have found their 'natural' home in the Republican Party (the GOP) and as such now have their hands on the tillers of state power. This is not altogether surprising, as I noted back in 2002; 'both the MMM and the CPK have close associations with elements of the American Republican Party and the British Conservative Party, and each movement finds adherents amongst white, working-class, lower-middle class males.'[189]

---

[187] Whitehead, S. (2021) *Toxic Masculinity: Curing the Virus*. Luton: AG Books. P. 131.

[188] Whitehead, S. M. (2002) p. 68.

[189] Whitehead, S.M. (2002) p. 68.

No Longer Unassailable

Where the GOP is today, in terms of its overtly anti-feminist position and policies, can be traced back to the 1990s and the first organised responses by men to the rise of feminism and the rise of independent femininity: the gender revolution. Until the 90s, men didn't really take that much notice of women, at least as a powerful gender in their own right. Women, females, were marginalised, disempowered and, so the men assumed, controllable and under the patriarchal yoke. In other words, women were no threat to men's power, position and sense of maleness. Women didn't count and therefore men didn't feel obliged to include them in their power equations. As long as they gave women occasional mollifiers in terms of equal rights legislation, especially around work, education and marriage, and promoted a few to top positions in politics and industry, the men felt unassailable; confident that women were secured in their patriarchal box and for the most part, untroublesome. The men in power knew only too well that legislation can be changed. It can be given and it can be taken away. As long as men dominated politics and industry, certainly behind the throne if not always sitting on it, then they held all the aces – they were pretty much invulnerable. The non-negotiable point was that their male power must remain intact, their masculinity unthreatened – these had to remain undiminished, if not always unquestioned.

In every respect, but especially politically, at the beginning of the twenty-first century women were living in what some feminists have described as a 'sexist misogynistic wasteland',[190] excluded from the masculinist empire and its decision-making processes, just as they had been throughout history – a situation that men didn't plan on changing any time soon. Women were visible and appreciated primarily as sexual or maternal subjects, their traditional femininity defined by men, scripted in religious texts and signified in language, image and culture. But once women found a united voice and become publicly and politically active, thereby putting real pressure on men and their patriarchal attitudes, men's ambivalence and patronising attitude towards them disappeared fast. From the turn of the millennium onwards, women started to take note of what it cost them to be quiet and to acquiesce to male dominance and maleist attitudes: especially to remain silent in the face of male abuse, harassment, rape and murder. The radical feminists of the 1970s had always warned that beneath the visible surface of male patronisation, institutional sexism, rape, murder

---

[190] https://thenewfeminist.co.uk/2022/04/why-the-2000s-was-a-sexist-wasteland/

and sexual harassment of women was an ocean of hatred for women. The term 'femicide'[191] started to be used more often, and countries with some of the highest rates of hate-killings of females were pressured by feminist activists to classify femicide as a hate crime;[192] Mexico, Peru, Argentina and Canada being just some of the countries where women took to publicly protesting against femicide and the numerous disappearances of women.[193] The visible universality of crimes against women grew dramatically in the public consciousness once social media took off in 2003. In April 2004, the March for Women's Lives in Washington D.C. had a record 1.15 million participants.[194] In 2006, the phrase 'MeToo' began to be used by women who'd been sexually abused and raped by men, and by 2017 had become a viral social media movement encouraging millions of women to publicise their experiences of men's violence.[195] Suddenly, there were fewer places or indeed opportunities for male abusers to hide. Every man was now required to look at his behaviour, whether abusive towards women or not. From here on, men had no excuses. They could no longer hide behind religious, gender or cultural discourses nor claim ignorance as to the effects of their behaviour towards women. Women were telling men how they felt and the accusations stung, not least because men knew them to be true.

---

[191] https://theconversation.com/femicide-many-countries-around-the-world-are-making-the-killing-of-women-a-specific-crime-heres-why-its-needed-227526

For detailed discussion, see Dawson, M. and Vega, M.V. (eds) (2023) *The Routledge International Handbook on Femicide and Feminicide*. London: Routledge. https://www.who.int/news-room/fact-sheets/detail/violence-against-women

[192] https://pmc.ncbi.nlm.nih.gov/articles/PMC10795990/

[193] https://www.theguardian.com/world/2017/jan/21/womens-march-protests-history-suffragettes-iceland-poland https://www.jstor.org/stable/10.3998/mpub.11953892.7?seq=7

[194] https://now.org/about/history/history-of-marches-and-mass-actions/#:~:text=the%20federal%20courts.-,2004%20March%20for%20Women's%20Lives,largest%20protest%20in%20U.S.%20history. Also, https://www.aljazeera.com/gallery/2024/11/26/thousands-rally-across-the-world-calling-for-end-to-violence-against-women https://giwps.georgetown.edu/violence-targeting-women-in-politics-10-countries-to-watch-in-2022/

[195] https://www.verywellmind.com/what-is-the-metoo-movement-4774817#:~:text=New%20York%20City%20women's%20advocate,and%20adoption%20across%20social%20media.

However, like any catalyst, the impact was not only one way. In demanding they change, many men responded to women by going in entirely the opposite direction, becoming openly misogynistic, especially on social media. Though frankly these diehard misogynists didn't need much encouragement; such men were always going to hit back at women once they stopped playing the patriarchal game and stood up for themselves.

In waking up to the new gender equation presented by a strident, capable, vocal womanhood, men were forced to look more closely at themselves as men and at their masculinity. None of which was welcomed nor comfortable for the male species. It was a bit like a junior female employee in a large corporation gate-crashing the male-dominated directors' meeting wherein she precisely and tellingly confronts them with their failings and how they need to change.

A United Front

In building a united masculinist front against all women, anti-feminist men have found it useful to enjoin with some unlikely partners. For example, what we've witnessed with the CPK in America, where it has morphed into the Christian Right (a dominant, powerful religious/political coalition of anti-feminists and anti-LGBTQ+, now fully embraced by the GOP) is mirrored around the world: Jewish fundamentalists in Israel; Islamic fundamentalists everywhere; and patriarchs in Buddhism, Hinduism, Catholicism, indeed all religions historically dominated by men. Whatever their religious belief and no matter how devotedly they follow it and differentiate it from other religious beliefs, all the millions of traditional males embracing the radical versions of these religions have a common cause – they hate feminists and they recognise any independent feminine woman to be their greatest enemy, their greatest threat; their ideological and personal emasculator.

The burgeoning gender revolution, while still not recognised as such by most people, was by the mid-noughties really stirring the pot of masculinity and churning up some very contrasting responses from men. Foremost in this bubbling pot was the concept of masculinity itself: most men innocently imagined, if they thought of masculinity at all, that it was something fixed, predictable, inevitable, maybe ordained by some Higher Power and pretty much the same the world over. In other words, stable and biologically determined. None of which turned out to be true. Because by then sociologists like myself had already spent at least thirty years studying men and masculinities and deduced some fascinating truths about it. For example, its contingency, insecurities, cultural specificity, multiplicity, fluidity, how it relates to sexuality and language, and how it impacts on, for example, men's mental health and emotional well-being.

The average guy in the street would not be expected to know any of this; he was preoccupied with being a man, belonging to the community of men, and finding ways of demonstrating his masculinity in whatever way he deemed most positive, protective and beneficial to his identity as a masculine subject. For him all this attention on his maleness would have been a rude awakening. Throughout millennia men had never been required to question who they were as men, as masculine subjects, to reflect on how they came to be men, to think about masculinity critically or even to recognise when they were performing it. This was why I couldn't mention the word 'masculinity' to my doctoral interviewees – it would have been akin to poisoning the clear water of their untroubled male subjectivity. Of course, by the time I undertook my PhD, all that clear water was starting to get churned up, disrupted, and eventually became poisoned anyway. The gender revolution was doing that.

It is also instructive to reflect on the transference of language and labels. Not that long ago, 'left and right' in political terms signalled 'communism vs capitalism' and 'socialist vs liberal economics'. All that has changed and very quickly. Not surprisingly, the various political groups responding to the rise of feminism inevitably polarised into the pro-feminists and the anti-feminists, woke and non-woke, progressive and conservative. Now we see Putin aligning politically not just with Xi Jinping but with Trump's GOP, their common ground being their anti-feminist, anti-LGBTQ+ stance. The economic contest between opposing ideologies and the 'great power competition' between US, Russia and China hasn't gone away, but it is no longer the only global contest. The emergent contest, the gender revolution, cuts across traditional national identities, politics and eternal obsessions with geopolitical hegemony.

> *The many millions of women with independent femininity have more in common with each other, no matter their nationality, religion, or race, than they have with the men who supposedly love them, hate them or attempt to have control over them.*

The gender revolution is about much more than Putin's empire building, Xi Jinping's desire for control over large swathes of East and South East Asia, or Trump's MAGA complex; such global contests are nothing new – they have long been a part of the human story. But the gender revolution is different. Why? Because it exists to change the historic gender status quo and is therefore a direct threat to those men rooted to the old gender order. Only the gender revolution offers a direct threat to men's power, which is why, globally, the array of forces now opposed to feminism and feminists is formidable; even greater than that which Russia, China, the USA, the Western democracies and large parts of the rest of world presented during the Cold War (1945-1991). Traditional adversaries find they now speak the same language when it comes to feminism, LGBTQ+ rights, identity politics and the culture wars. These voices of the men in power, no matter whether they arise from a democratic or authoritarian state, harmonise in chorusing the threat of feminism, the dangers inherent in liberalised gender identities, and the risks to them personally and politically in allowing women true independence of femininity.

But nuclear missile systems, weaponised drones and massed armies are of little use in this conflict. And anyway, the male protagonists still haven't realised who is opposing them. In their maleist ignorance they imagine it to be the radical feminism of the 70s and 80s, when in reality it is now a large slice of the world's population calling these men out and demanding change.

The Masculinity Responses

The feminist notion that the 'personal is political' is powerfully illustrated when we examine how masculinity has been variously impacted over the past few decades by the rise of women, the universality of independent femininity and the gender revolution. These contrasting responses are, however, not biological but discursive; which means they can and do change even while having the power to influence men's thoughts and behaviour.

> *'We must not imagine a world of discourse divided between accepted discourse and excluded discourse, or between dominant discourse and the dominated one; but as a multiplicity of discursive elements than can come into play in various strategies... Discourse transmits and produces power; it reinforces it, but also undermines and exposes it, renders it fragile and makes it possible to thwart it.'*[196]

---

[196] Michel Foucault (1984), quoted in Ramazanoglu, C. (ed) (1993) *Up Against Foucault*. London: Routledge. P. 19.

Men In Crisis

Masculinity discourses may be proliferating in the twenty-first century but back in the 80s and 90s the only time you'd have come across any media discussion of masculinity, or even seen the word in print, would have been in terms of it being in crisis. By the mid-90s the male crisis was regular mainstream news. No matter that throughout history there had been periodic eruptions of 'male crises', especially when it came to concerns over men's fitness for war,[197] this time the crisis felt real for a great many folk, generating heated media debates, a host of articles, interviews and books. It even produced one of the most renowned films about men and masculinity: *Fight Club*, released in 1999.

> '*Fight Club* is, by and large, an effective film that surrealistically describes the status of the American male at the end of the twentieth century: disenchanted, unfulfilled, castrated, and looking for a way out… In an era where men do not have missions, in the urban wilderness, what is there to hunt? To dominate? To kill?'[198]

Maybe in answer to the above existential question posed to American males, it didn't take long for that country's male leaders to find someone to kill: following 9/11 they were embarked on wars in both Afghanistan and Iraq. This tells you something about men and their masculinity; they're very quick to cry "crisis" if they perceive any threat to their manliness – and such threats can, in reality, only come from the opposite sex: women, the reason being that masculinity exists, at least traditionally, in opposition to femininity. It shows that the relationship between men and their masculinity is tenuous at best and in constant need of reassurance, and that one way that men achieve masculine reassurance is by having power over women.

---

[197] For example, the Boy Scouts of America were formed in 1910, precisely to create a new generation of 'masculine males'. Thirty years later, Hitler feared that the menfolk of Germany were not tough enough to fight another world war. While in recent years similar concerns have been expressed by Vladimir Putin and Xi Jinping regarding the prevalence of 'soft and emasculated males' willing to fight and die for their country. See Whitehead, S.M. (2002) for discussion, Chapter 2. Also, https://www.brandeis.edu/writing-program/write-now/2020-2021/dragunoff-alex/index.html https://www.bbc.com/news/world-asia-china-55926248

[198] From Whitehead, S.M. (2002) P.49-50.

The other way is through violence. Acting similarly to a narcotic, violence gives men an instant shot of masculine validation. History shows how easily and willingly male leaders slip into escalating violence as a response to political uncertainties and incomprehension as to true realities and intents; all messaged as a need to 'kick ass', 'show who's top dog', and 'shock and awe'. However, invariably lurking behind all that macho posturing lies something altogether more basic – fear. As war historian A.J.P. Taylor notes;

> 'Wars in fact have sprung more from apprehension than from a lust for war or for conquest. Paradoxically, many of the European wars were started by a threatened power which had nothing to gain by war and much to lose.'[199]

Unfortunately, like narcotics, violence also has withdrawal systems, as millions of ex-soldiers, from Vietnam to Afghanistan, WWI to WWII, know only too well.

By the turn of the millennium, the crisis of masculinity thesis had become a worldwide staple discourse informing societal understandings of modern men, triggering something akin to a global moral panic over the state of males of all ages and types; encapsulating concerns over males and health, crime, education, employment and family life. According to many commentators of the day, we were now in a 'postfeminist era' with hapless men becoming the 'disposable sex'; 'stiffed'; 'feminized'; 'emasculated' and trapped 'in a major male identity crisis' requiring them to 'reassess their masculinity' and 'facing a bleak, unforgiving future'.[200]

Despite all this fervent and feverish male angst and handwringing, as one feminist shrewdly observed at the time: *'The meanings and fantasies accompanying the equation of men and power are largely undisturbed'*.[201]

And of course – as we were to quickly find out – she was right.

Male Fundamentalism

Looking back, one can see how quickly men gathered themselves together, formed ranks, circled the wagons and fixed bayonets once women started to rise up in number and the gender revolution picked up pace. Having

---

[199] Taylor, A.J.P. (2024) *How Wars Begin and End.* London: Lume Books. P. 10

[200] See Whitehead, S.M. (2002) Chapter 2.

[201] Segal, L. (1999) *Why Feminism? Gender, Psychology, Politics.* Cambridge: Polity. P. 161.

been rudely awoken from their long historic sleep during which they may have dreamt masculine dreams but certainly didn't learn more about their masculine selves, men's first response was incredulity mixed with fear: look what is happening to us! How can we survive? We are being emasculated by feminists, by women! We will lose everything! It is not natural! It is against God's law!

History shows men didn't lose everything – instead, and predictably, they simply resisted. The male identity crisis disappeared almost as fast as it arose. At time of writing, with right-wing anti-feminist governments in power in many countries, including the USA, there is no longer any talk of a male crisis, only direct threats to women encapsulated in aggressive macho statements such as "your body, my choice".[202]

Trump and the GOP are now explicitly and unapologetically male fundamentalists. They are no longer simply opposing feminists, LGBTQ+ and the so-called 'woke', they are *opposing all women*. Perhaps they recognise the emergence of independent femininity across the USA and globally? I've no idea, but we should at least recognise how resistance to feminism has now expanded and solidified to become resistance to women as a gender group; certainly, women with independent femininity, which is likely to be the majority.

I define male fundamentalism as follows:

> *Male fundamentalism is an unapologetic explicitly anti-female, misogynistic position adopted by men. It transcends religious affiliation, culture, nationality, race, ethnicity and other identity variables. It privileges heterosexuality and male power, and assumes an unchallengeable and inevitable biological (and/or) religious basis to men's supremacy over women. Male fundamentalists believe in the right to control women in the public and private spheres through the maintenance of an inflexible gender binary, reinforced by a judicial system and, if necessary, physical force.*

Examples of organised, systemised, institutionalised and extremist male fundamentalism in the world today would include the Taliban in Afghanistan,[203] the Shia radicals of Iran[204] and the Wahhabi movement of

---

[202] https://www.theguardian.com/commentisfree/2024/nov/13/your-body-my-choice-maga-men

[203] In January 2025, Malala Yousafzai informed Muslim leaders in Pakistan that "the Taliban in Afghanistan do not see women as human beings". https://www.bbc.com/news/articles/c70qz9ly1eko

Saudi Arabia, all of which promote and install gender apartheid in their regimes. Additional countries imposing some aspect of gender apartheid include Malaysia, Indonesia and Pakistan, along with numerous countries in the Middle East.[205]

More randomised, dispersed male fundamentalists would include incels, discussed below; individual men adherents of Christian, Jewish and Muslim Orthodox religious discourses; and those men supporting extreme right-wing political policies which are anti-feminist, anti-LGBTQ+, anti-choice and anti-inclusion – i.e. many male GOP supporters in the USA and right-wing political supporters elsewhere around the world.

All of these groups and the individual men who adhere to male fundamentalism are fully prepared to protect male privilege and patriarchal structures in any way they see necessary, including institutionalised and random violence against women and any of their allies. The physical and psychological threat to females posed by male fundamentalists is very real and needs to be challenged, globally. While its most obvious manifestation is the explicit gender apartheid now being carried out in Afghanistan, Iran and Saudi Arabia, the actual form such apartheid takes may well differ from country to country, regime to regime.

One potential consequence of the gender revolution and the global rise in independent femininity is that other countries with male fundamentalist leaders may take note of how the Taliban, Iranian and Saudi Arabian patriarchies operate against women and decide to copy them. For example, by reducing females' educational opportunities, work opportunities, communication opportunities, even physical movement – confining them to the home and under the control of a male 'guardian'. Also, by putting pressure on women to marry, conceive and thereby increase birth rates. One might say we are a long way from such a situation in America and other 'liberal democracies' (e.g. in parts of East Europe) and even in authoritarian

---

[204] https://theconversation.com/how-irans-government-has-weaponized-sexual-violence-against-women-who-dare-to-resist-253791

[205] https://endgenderapartheid.today/   https://www.theguardian.com/global-development/2024/oct/09/what-is-gender-apartheid-activists-international-law-women-girls-rights-afghanistan-iran   https://en.wikipedia.org/wiki/Gender_apartheid   https://www.amnesty.org/en/latest/news/2024/06/gender-apartheid-must-be-recognized-international-law/ . Iran has set up 'mental health clinics' to 'treat' women who refuse to wear the hijab and as an attempt to squash the 'Woman, Life, Freedom' uprising which started in 2022. https://apple.news/A9keaOejLSB-Ovj4ix9z2iw

states such as Russia and China, but its wise not to underestimate the anger of male fundamentalists, their fear of independent femininity, and their intention to roll back the gender revolution, especially if they are in control of governments.[206]

The incel is one example of male fundamentalism that has gathered a lot of global attention since the first incel attack, in California in 2014. Since, then a rabid and vehemently misogynistic online 'community' has arisen, dominated by male heterosexuals (of various races, religions and nationalities) and targeting women, both via online hate messaging, trolling, stalking, and in physical attacks. The incel, or involuntary celibate, believe women '*are unjustly denying them sexual or romantic attention*'.[207]

> "Women are the cause of our suffering. They are the ones who unjustly made our lives a living hell. We need to focus more on our hatred of women. Hatred is power."[208]

For the vast majority of people confronted with the bizarre rationale and terrifying behaviour of the incel, it is like being plunged into a dystopian Margaret Atwood novel, with yourself as a reluctant participant, the difference being that this is not fiction but reality. Can the incel ever be cured of his anger, hatred and returned to live peacefully in civilised society? Not through imprisonment, which is where a great many of them will end up. These men are psychologically damaged and that damage is being fuelled daily by social media, on platforms such as X and Reddit. The incel is one of the key reasons for the growing gender divergence, though perhaps not an entirely unexpected response from disenfranchised men to the rise of independent femininity.

Relatedly, also becoming more common are instances of men randomly attacking women in the street, for example – women being punched in the face by strangers while walking in New York and other American cities; such attacks likely intended to instil fear in all women while making prosecution

---

[206] In rolling back the gender revolution, and as part of a general conservative backlash, male fundamentalists will include DEI programmes, thus attempting to 'end the push for greater diversity' across business, education, and general society. There are already many examples of this happening in the USA https://www.theguardian.com/business/2025/jan/06/mcdonalds-diversity-programs?CMP=Share_iOSApp_Other

[207] See Whitehead, S. (2021) p.41-42.

[208] Ibid. p. 40.

of the male perpetrator harder to pursue.[209] Such actions also illustrate how, throughout history, men have demonstrated a remarkable capacity for violence and hatred, no matter how illogical. Further confirmation is given in the global rise of mass killings by men and there is some justification for linking the male heterosexual incels with those men (also usually heterosexual) who demonstrate hatred of all society and enact 'revenge against society' attacks on total strangers.

> *'There can be no doubt – patriarchy, misogyny, domestic abuse and mass murder are associated, and have been for a long time. Emerging empirical research further highlights misogynistic attitudes are outwardly expressed in diverse forms of extremism, such as far-right extremism, jihadism, and 'misogynistic incels'.*[210]

At time of writing there have been at least nine mass killings and attacks in China during 2024, three more than in the entire previous decade.[211]

---

[209] https://www.nytimes.com/2024/04/12/nyregion/new-york-city-random-attacks-women.html   https://www.cbsnews.com/newyork/news/nyc-women-randomly-attacked-punched-slapped/ .   https://www.cesifo.org/DocDL/cesifo1_wp7009.pdf This is not a situation unique to New York, Dallas, Chicago, Philadelphia or Los Angeles. In London, 75% of women have reported being subjected to harassment or violence in public. https://assets.publishing.service.gov.uk/media/5a81bd72ed915d74e33ffcd8/Infrastructure-Cities-briefing-note.pdf?t In Latin America, 6 in 10 women reported being physically harassed while using public transport. In Port Moresby, Papua New Guinea, 90% of women have experienced some form of sexual violence on public transport. More than 83% of Egyptian women have been harassed on Cairo's streets. Only 12% of women in Lima feel safe in the city. Women 'who looked like feminists' (e.g. have short hair) have been attacked in public in South Korea. https://www.theguardian.com/world/2024/nov/15/4b-south-korea-feminist-movement-donald-trump-election-backlash?CMP=Share_iOSApp_Other Groups of local men have been reported attacking foreign women in Hanoi https://vn.usembassy.gov/rise-in-attacks-on-foreign-women/

[210] https://discovery.ucl.ac.uk/id/eprint/10185280/1/A%20Common%20Psychology%20of%20Male%20Violence%20%20Assessing%20the%20Effects%20of%20Misogyny%20on%20Intentions%20to%20Engage%20in%20Violent%20Extremism%20%20Interpersonal%20Violence%20and%20Suppo.pdf?t https://www.tandfonline.com/doi/full/10.1080/09546553.2023.2292723?t

[211] https://apnews.com/article/china-vehicle-car-knife-attack-b1534d572f0f2b34f0d2f1bec109a693

Similar attacks, usually but not always as mass shootings, have become commonplace in the USA over recent decades while also occurring in many other countries including Norway, Australia, New Zealand, Thailand, Canada, Tasmania, France, Belgium and the UK. Aside from the gender commonality are the religious, fascist and racist ideologies of many of these perpetrators.

While it should be acknowledged that hatred towards women has been a motivator for the murder and rape of women since time immemorial, not all incels are violent, even if all are psychologically prone to misogyny. They are, however, a significant part of the 'manosphere', a global online 'community' of interconnected misogynistic groups, which also encompasses 'Men Going Their Own Way', 'Men's Rights Activists' and 'Pick-up Artists'.[212] Male representatives of the manosphere are increasingly finding themselves in the news for all the wrong reasons, an example being mixed martial arts fighter Conor McGregor; in December 2024 he was ordered by a Dublin civil court jury to pay over €250,000 to Nikita Hand, who it is claimed he "brutally raped and battered".

> 'This case has prompted calls for a rethink of how society interacts with power, wealth and a 'manosphere' intent on pushing its own notions of masculinity.'[213]

In examining the more extreme and lethal responses by men to the gender revolution, we should distinguish between the acts of violence perpetrated against women by male fundamentalists – which can be defined as terrorism against women and LGBTQ+ people – and the 'everyday' violence that women around the world suffer from men, especially in the home. While the consequences are the same – terror, death, harm or trauma – the origins of the violence are different. The male fundamentalist will draw on a variety of discourses to 'justify' his violence against women – religion, masculine power, culture – or simply because he fears women's growing power as a gender group. Consequently, in one respect this type of violence is not personal against the woman or female – any woman or female will suffice as a victim, even children – e.g. the Southport UK stabbings in August 2024.[214]

---

[212] https://en.wikipedia.org/wiki/Manosphere https://www.internetmatters.org/hub/news-blogs/what-is-the-manosphere-and-why-is-it-a-concern/

[213] https://www.theguardian.com/society/2024/dec/02/conor-mcgregor-verdict-manosphere-masculinity

[214] https://news.sky.com/story/southport-stabbings-suspect-faces-separate-terror-charge-after-ricin-and-al-qaeda-manual-found-at-home-13243980

By contrast, the vast majority of men who are violent towards women, for example Conor McGregor, and the 51 Frenchmen accused of the rape of Gisele Pelicot, are not on a political quest to defend patriarchy but are simply taking advantage of an individual woman's physical weakness, vulnerability and availability so as to satisfy their lust, anger, frustration or ameliorate their mental state. This is the 'stranger danger' that all women face, but which men rarely recognise.[215]

All acts of violence against women are terrorising, but it is the male fundamentalist who should be declared the terrorist as he is acting with deliberate if not strategic intent and as part of a politicised entity that has a declared objective of crushing women's independence from men, along with the intent to kill and harm women if they resist his impositions.

We also need to recognise that this is not about woke or anti-woke politics – though they make for convenient if reductive, labels. It is fundamentally about women's rights and men's power over them. The male fundamentalist will only be content when women are back where they were in the 1950s, metaphorically (and maybe literally) wearing skirts, not trousers. The fear that such men have about the loss of their hegemony, patriarchal dividends and male privileges is palpable and it is that fear that is dangerous and threatening to women everywhere and to all those who support women's independence from men and their right to live without fear of male violence.

Traditional Masculinity

This is the most common type of masculinity. It doesn't dominate in every community, culture or organisation, but when examining men as a global species then traditional masculinity is what prevails. As I explore in this section, traditional masculinity includes quite an eclectic mix of attitudes and behaviours, ranging from the closeted homophobe to the unapologetic chauvinist. Some men with traditional masculinity may even consider themselves liberal allies of women, others will be on the edges of misogyny. What is common among all men with traditional masculinity is an inability to shake off the notion that (heterosexual) men are the 'naturally' dominant species and that their dominance over women is an unalterable 'fact of life'. Therefore, in their minds, while it is fine to allow women more equality and freedom, it is not so fine to allow women to lead, dominate, and exercise power, especially over men.

---

[215] https://apple.news/AQqlosHafTKKm1eViVAIW-Q

I define traditional masculinity (aka hegemonic or toxic masculinity) as follows:

> 'A form of male behaviour and expression of male identity that seeks to reinforce men's power and patriarchal values. Based on characteristics such as competition, ambition, self-reliance, physical strength, aggression and homophobia, the image that is perpetrated celebrates physical toughness, the endurance of hardships, aggressiveness, a rugged heterosexuality, and unemotional logic.'[216]

Traditional masculinity is a way of being a man and expressing manliness, drawing on the following dominant discourses or value systems;

1. Homophobia/transphobia
2. Patriarchy
3. Emotional impediment and reticence (also stoicism)
4. Compulsory heterosexuality
5. Rigid gender binary – gender/sex roles and a gendered public and private spheres
6. Exercise of power and accompanying demonstration of physical strength

While globally the majority of men will not succumb to male fundamentalism, most will be touched by the discourses informing traditional masculinity. That is why in 2018 the American Psychological Association (APA) issued a statement '*advising psychologists on recognizing masculine ideology when working with men and boys.*'

> 'Traditional masculinity ideology includes elements of anti-femininity, achievement, eschewal of the appearance of weakness, and adventure, risk and violence'.[217]

Traditional masculinity is toxic, hegemonic and dangerous to women, men and children, whatever their intersectional identity. Indeed, most laypeople will recognise it as 'toxic masculinity' a term that I have helped promote in

---

[216] Whitehead, S. (2021) p. 30

[217] https://www.apa.org/monitor/2019/01/ce-corner https://www.apa.org/about/policy/boys-men-practice-guidelines.pdf

my writings since 2013, and which went viral in 2016.[218] This performance of male identity has many layers and expressions, but at its heart is a capacity for aggression and violence, especially towards women.

The scale of men's violences against women that has been recorded through history is staggering if not beyond comprehension, and yet most remains unrecorded. It includes the random, the opportunistic and the premeditated. Just how far 'ordinary' men can go in their violences towards women and girls is powerfully revealed in single examples, such as, at time of writing, the horrific sexual atrocities perpetrated on Tigrayan women by Ethiopian and Eritean soldiers;[219] the systematic rape and mutilation of women at the Nova music festival, Israel, by Hamas on 7th October 2024;[220] and the growing number of reports of sexual and gender-based violence against Palestinian women and girls by Israeli soldiers during the current Gaza war.[221] These and similar acts of sexual violence are not explained by war so much as by toxic masculinity. War simply provides men with an opportunity for culturally sanctioned sexual violence, and is increasingly doing so as part of a larger 'war on women'.[222]

The men who rape, abuse, traffic women and children, operate criminal gangs, carry out domestic abuse and perpetrate physical, emotional and psychological violence against women, will have traditional (toxic) masculinity and indeed will draw on traditional gender discourses to try and justify their behaviour. They are certainly not allied to feminists or LGBTQ+ people, and in fact are a potential danger to all of society, not just to women but also to other men. The reason is that they assume violence to be a natural if not useful way of men 'resolving' conflict and in many instances, an acceptable means of achieving their aims and ambitions.

There are many aspects to traditional/toxic masculinity which cannot be explored fully here, though it should be noted that not only is this way of

---

[218] See Whitehead, S. et al, (2013) and Whitehead, S. (2021)

[219] https://www.theguardian.com/global-development/2025/jun/30/sexual-violence-tigray-women-abuse-gang-rape-ethiopia-eritrea?CMP=Share_iOSApp_Other

[220] https://www.bbc.com/news/world-middle-east-67629181

[221] https://en.wikipedia.org/wiki/Sexual_and_gender-based_violence_against_Palestinians_during_the_Gaza_war

[222] https://www.theguardian.com/global-development/2024/oct/23/un-women-report-civilian-deaths-children-war-zones-2023-access-healthcare

being a danger to others, especially women, it is also harmful to those men who exhibit it and who, as the APA notes, 'draw on masculine ideology' in their self-creation of maleness. Certainly, the mental health of traditionally minded men is shown to be less robust than in progressive men:

> 'It takes more courage to reveal insecurities than to hide them, more strength to relate to people than to dominate them, more 'manhood' to abide by thought-out principles rather than blind reflex. Toughness is in the soul and spirit, not in muscles and an immature mind.'[223]

Some men may draw on 'male pride and strength' discourses to 'justify' their traditional/toxic masculinity (e.g. Andrew Tate) while others may use more intellectualist arguments (e.g. Jordan Petersen).[224] Whatever the source of their 'evidence' or the rhetoric used to promote it, the objective is the same; to counter women's growing independence and restore a traditional gender order with men firmly placed at the top.

In comparing the male fundamentalist with a man who adheres to traditional masculinity, though the former will certainly have a traditional masculinity, he's taken it a step further than most traditionally minded men would, which is to treat women as 'the enemy', and to be especially hostile to any woman presenting an independent mindset, attitude or resistance to male power – obviously feminists, but also LGBTQ+ people, indeed any individual not prepared to acquiesce to patriarchal demands. In contrast, many men with traditional masculinity are not necessarily politically active against women, violent against women, nor see women as the enemy. Though their masculine sense of self draws on discourses and beliefs that serve to render and position women as the Other – secondary, subordinate, subject to men's authority and diminished – such men may not realise they are sexist and thereby a threat to women's independent femininity. Again, men's lack of self-awareness plays a large part in creating this gender divergence. However, if women subsequently challenge male authority then it can potentially generate a violent response from such men, either in the

---

[223] https://www.thegrayarea.com.au/heretohear/mental-health-the-modern-man?t

[224] https://theconversation.com/from-andrew-tate-to-jordan-peterson-a-phoney-zero-sum-game-argument-sits-at-the-heart-of-anti-feminist-backlash-194665#:~:text=The%20arguments%20put%20forward%20by%20Tate%20and,be%20physically%20strong%20and%20seek%20resources%20and

home or in the street. They can experience women's expressiveness and power as a direct and very personal threat to who they are as men.

At time of writing, there have been eruptions of explicit traditional masculinity backlashes against women in India, South Korea, Ecuador, China, Poland, Myanmar, Philippines, Venezuela, Cuba, Algeria, Belarus, Kuwait, Sudan, Yemen, Mexico, Haiti, Dominican Republic, Pakistan, South Africa, Congo, Egypt, Kenya, Morocco, Honduras, Brazil, Russia, Iran, Afghanistan and Chad.[225] The harsh fact is that no woman is 100% safe from male violence anywhere, though the safest countries for women are consistently shown to be Denmark, Switzerland, Sweden, Iceland, Norway and Finland.

Progressive Masculinity

If all that appears rather depressing, and it is, then there is also global evidence of men becoming more civilised and less violent. Or at least not so tempted *en masse* to rejoice in wholesale slaughter, genocide, human sacrifice and grotesque and bloody public executions; e.g. indulge in the everyday orgies of sadism which have hitherto defined the human experience. This is a 'civilising process' first noticed by German sociologist Norbert Elias in 1939 and more recently finely analysed by Canadian-American sociologist, Stephen Pinker, in his book, *The Better Angels of Our Nature* (2010).

The notion that 'humanity' (Pinker really means men) is becoming less not more violent – even more empathetic – is, as Pinker acknowledges, counter-intuitive at the very least if not readily rejected by 'common-sense'. Yet the evidence is compelling and Pinker examines the full extent of it. One of his conclusions is that we have the rise of feminism and the women's rights movements of the past seven or so decades to thank for this civilising of the male species.

> *'Studies from 1970 to 1995 show that college-age men and women… had increasingly progressive attitudes towards women. In fact, the men of the early 1990s had attitudes that were more feminist than those of the women of the 1970s… Despite anecdote-driven claims that women have made no progress because of a "backlash"*

---

[225] https://www.hrw.org/news/2023/03/07/global-backlash-against-womens-rights https://counteringbacklash.org/update/countering-gender-backlash-in-africa-and-asia/ https://ejournals.bib.uni-wuppertal.de/index.php/sws/article/view/64/366 https://www.cesifo.org/DocDL/cesifo1_wp7009.pdf

> *against feminism, data show that the country's [USA] attitudes have become inexorably more progressive. Western cultures default point of view has increasingly become unisex. We are all feminists now.*'[226]

Clearly, 'we are not all feminists now' and likely never will be. But nevertheless, Pinker (and Elias) are correct in identifying a trend, at least among women and a growing minority of men, and that is towards progressive gender and sexual attitudes. This process, accompanied by what Pinker describes as a 'reorientation of moral and legal systems so that they could be justified from a viewpoint that is not specific to men', can be seen as evidence for a global shift towards a feminisation of society, central to which, in my view, is independent femininity and, de facto, the gender revolution.

But as detailed in this chapter, not all men are part of this hopeful story. Only a global minority, albeit a significant and influential minority. These are men with a reflective, empathetic character. They are liberal, supportive of DEIJ initiatives, anti-racist, pro-LGBTQ+, even adopting a pro-feminist position and allying with women seeking gender justice. Such men have embraced a progressive masculinity, which I define as follows:

> 'A man with progressive masculinity believes in equality for women, is pro-LGBTQ+; considers that all societies must challenge male abuse, male violence and patriarchal values; does not seek to present himself as physically challenging to others, especially women; is an ally to women with independent femininity and is not threatened by such women; and supports the education of males away from physically and psychologically damaging behaviours.'[227]

There are twenty primary and secondary indicators of progressive masculinity:

The Ten Primary Indicators

1. He does not feel threatened by women's power or desire for independence

---

[226] Pinker, S. (2012) *The Better Angels of Our Nature: The Decline of Violence in History and its Causes.* London: Penguin. P. 403. Also, Elias, N. (1939/2000) *The Civilizing Process: Sociogentic and Psychogentic Investigations.* Cambridge, Mass.: Blackwell.

[227] See Whitehead, S. (2021) Chapter Four, for elaboration and examples.

2. Feminist: supports LGBTQ+ rights and the MeToo movement
3. Liberal-minded and open to alternative cultural expressions
4. Anti-racist
5. Reflective, self-aware, able to recognise and express his emotions positively
6. Negotiates and shares child-care duties with partner
7. Negotiates and shares household duties with partner (may be househusband)
8. Pro-choice (abortion and birth control)
9. Approaches intimate relationships from the standpoint of equality and equity
10. Masculinity not threatened by partners with higher professional status or earning power

The Ten Secondary Indicators

1. College/university educated
2. Seeks personal improvement (emotionally and intellectually)
3. Ambitious but also aims for a good work-life balance
4. Not avidly following any single religion but possibly spiritual
5. Can articulate his feelings and thoughts
6. Not prone to outbursts of aggression or violence
7. Comfortable with new technology
8. Considers himself a global citizen with an international mindedness
9. Has developed emotional bonds and friendship networks with straight and gay men
10. Uses social media but not in an aggressive or predatory manner

I consider the most critical variable to be the first: *the man is either a declared feminist or he is comfortable with, and therefore unthreatened by, the power that women are acquiring and expressing today.* He would also be fully supportive of women's independent femininity.[228] All the primary indicators are non-negotiable and must be present in the man's attitude, sense of self and practices. The secondary indicators will not exist in every progressive man nor necessarily be consistent over time. Nor am I suggesting that all men with progressive masculinity are pacifists. But taken as a whole, these twenty indicators offer a realistic portrait of the key variables intersecting to form progressive masculinity in a man.

The number of men, globally, with a progressive masculine identity is difficult to quantify, but it would start with the 5–10% who openly identify as pro-feminists, this figure varying greatly depending on the country – though not all these men will be necessarily be active in promoting women's rights and challenging patriarchal practices. While pro-feminist men may not account for the majority of men with progressive masculinity, they are certainly in the majority when it comes to promoting feminist activities. There are now pro-feminist workshops on gender equality led by men (and women) and being delivered to boys and men in numerous countries, including; USA, UK, China, South Africa, Spain, El Salvador, Australia, India, Canada, Brazil and across Scandinavia. Such activities are supported by, amongst others, UNESCO, European Institute for Gender Equality, UN Women, Cynara, The Good Men Project, NOMAS and White Ribbon.[229]

As stated above, the key factor in progressive masculinity is not so much the man declaring he's a pro-feminist, but that he *does not feel threatened by women's independent femininity and the growing power of women.* In other words, his masculine self is not built on the edifice of male power over women and notions of male supremacy.

On that basis and informed by various studies, it is likely that the number of men with progressive masculinity rises to around 40% of men in countries such as the USA, Canada, UK, Australia, New Zealand and parts

---

[228] From Whitehead, S. et al. (2013) p.286.

[229] For example, https://www.cynara.co/trainingstore/engagingmen https://www.whiteribbon.org.uk/wrd24 https://www.engenderingindustries.org/resources/gender-equality-guides/engaging-men-gender-equality https://uniglobalunion.org/news/uni-africa-male-gender-equality-workshops/ https://goodmenproject.com/featured-content/better-to-lose-him-than-to-lose-me/?mc_cid=a478bb5e12&mc_eid=27f916f593 https://www.masculinitiesproject.org/transforming-men-workshops https://www.linkedin.com/company/man-up-wa/ https://nomas.org/ https://www.linkedin.com/in/harish-sadani-b821b410/ See also Whitehead, S. 2021, Chapters 9 and 10.

of Western Europe.[230] A 2023 survey of American adults showed 43% of men identifying as feminist, and there is little difference between Gen Z and Millennials in this identification,[231] while a global survey published at time of writing indicates 'that more than half the world's population identifies as feminist'.[232] As with women, a large percentage of men will decline the label 'feminist' while still advocating feminist values, equal rights for women and progressive masculinity.[233] However, no survey of a conceptual identity and political standpoint as volatile and emotive as 'feminist' can ever be totally accurate; it can only be an indicator. Much depends on who is asked, what is asked, when it is asked, and how it is asked. Nevertheless, it is clear that a large percentage of men would align with the values of diversity, inclusion, justice and equity, and this must include support for independent femininity. Compared to their brutal, sexist, vicious male ancestors, these men have indeed, become more civilised. Which in itself is a very welcome and positive change in men and therefore good for everyone else. And without doubt, the gender revolution is one of the key forces behind this 'civilising (of some men) process'.

More Masculinities?

Finally, an obvious question to ask is: how many more types of masculinity are there? And the answer is, no one knows. Every man is different, unique and living his solo life, just as is every woman and non-binary person. What I have described above are dominant patterns of male behaviour: attitudes, beliefs, values, responses and ways of thinking about gender identities, men and women, and ways of relating to them. All of which is both personal and

---

[230] https://www.maddyness.com/uk/2024/01/16/a-never-ending-struggle-new-data-reveals-that-antifeminists-outnumber-feminists-in-the-us/ https://www.kcl.ac.uk/news/uk-now-among-most-socially-liberal-of-countries https://www.mensjournal.com/news/study-major-decline-generation-z-men-identify-feminists https://aibm.org/commentary/no-young-men-are-not-turning-away-from-gender-equality/

[231] https://yougov.co.uk/international/articles/45362-who-feminist-west-2023-all-depends-question

[232] https://www.statista.com/statistics/312161/define-self-feminist-advocates-supports-equal-opportunities-women/

[233] https://yougov.co.uk/international/articles/45362-who-feminist-west-2023-all-depends-question

political. However, in the final analysis it comes back to a much simpler question for men: are you for or against women's independent femininity? And based on how men have responded thus far to women's rising power and assertiveness, we can categorise most men as either resisters or supporters, with both the respective camps containing avid resisters and avid supporters.

Of course, there will also be a lot of men who are 'don't knows'; who are still in the process of working it all out – the gender revolution – and its personal consequences for them. Though while they decide on which path to take (back to patriarchy or forward to independence for women) the gender revolution won't take a break. It is now speeding up fast, and I as examine in the next two chapters, so is the gender divergence and its consequences.

And then there are the many cultural and regional variations, all of which when taken together confirm the multiplicity of male identities. For example, in East Asia since the 90s, we have seen the emergence of a more androgynous masculinity, colloquially referred to as 'grass-eater' or 'herbivore' man. While this may indeed be a part-response to the rise of women, it is also linked to changing social patterns in Japan especially. Relatedly, and also across East Asia though emerging elsewhere, is the hikikomori male, in voluntary reclusion from all society. These male identities are also connected to the gender divergence while not yet forming a global masculinity.[234]

One thing for sure is that whatever the future of men and women, of all the genders, diversity will persist if not grow, as will people's desire for independence and freedom. This tells us that inclusion, equity and justice are vital if we are to avoid the end of sex and the further growing apart of women and men.

Concluding Observations

Men are in shock and have been for much of this century. Maybe not every man, but most. And how could they not be? Having spent millennia happily being men and doing manly things without scrutiny, being merely fixated on 'winning or losing', 'triumph or disaster', men suddenly found they were in the news not because of their deeds but because of their identity. Since around 2016, the whole world seems to have been talking about men and

---

[234] For discussion of different types of masculinity, including that encompassing 'grasseater' and hikikomori men, see Whitehead, S. (2021).

their identity, invariably discussing the evidence for – and consequences of – toxic masculinity; a term which for any gender sociologist is a useful simplification for what is actually happening in any man's head at any given time, but which for the average bloke can be a terrifying concept, similar in many ways to a virus. Have I got it? he might ask himself. And if I have, best not tell anyone.

Little wonder that many young men have responded to the gender revolution by heading deeper into the toxic masculine cave or rabbit hole. In retreat from their masculine insecurities, they remove themselves further away from modern society and certainly modern women. A process of voluntary male ghettoisation, the consequences of which are detailed in the final chapter. Not surprisingly, young males in the fraught process of being and becoming men may well listen to modern Pied Pipers of Hamlet; manosphere influencers like Andrew Tate, Adin Ross, Hamza Ahmed, Sneako and Jordan Petersen,[235] seducing naïve and insecure males deeper into the cave of no return, intoxicating them with dangerous and outdated notions of manliness. These and similar bad actors portray themselves as male mates against the 'woke', though when looked at more closely it turns out that 'woke' simply means any independent-minded female not prepared to suffer abuse and worse from any guy, e.g. their sister, girlfriend, partner or mother.

And who can blame women for finally resisting male power and the violence that inevitably accompanies it? For sure, men were quick to protest as soon as they realised the threat to their masculinity posed by feminists. How much more would men protest if they were subject to a global manicide[236] in the way that women are subject to a global femicide?

That a lot of guys out there are a threat to women is a given. But not all men. Most are simply struggling with the competing voices in their heads; the one urging them to be 'manly' and the other urging them to be compassionate and empathetic. Which voice wins out in the moment is

---

[235] https://theconversation.com/from-andrew-tate-to-jordan-peterson-a-phoney-zero-sum-game-argument-sits-at-the-heart-of-anti-feminist-backlash-194665
https://www.newsweek.com/andrew-tate-jordan-peterson-piers-morgan-reprehensible-1831947

https://www.theguardian.com/media/2025/mar/19/beyond-andrew-tate-the-imitators-who-help-promote-misogyny-online?CMP=Share_iOSApp_Other

[236] Manicide I define as the rampant and globalised murder of men by women. So, a fictional concept – not based in any reality.

influenced by many factors, most of which are to varying degrees outside the control of any man: upbringing, religion, culture, class, age, education, sexuality, health, peers, social media, and especially hope and opportunity.

Yet only when the man can *equate manliness with compassion and empathy for others* will the voices cease; until that happens he will be forever trapped between these two forces – one pulling him back the other pushing him forward.

And always in the background, behind the noise, is the ever-present fear: of failure, of not being manly enough, of showing weakness, of being ridiculed. Fear is the eternal leveller in the mind of every male who has ever lived and how each man deals with it, the threat behind the voices, tells you which voice he will listen to and act upon.

It is impossible to predict how any individual man will respond to the gender revolution, whether he will become an ally of women or an enemy, but what can be guaranteed is that every man lives with fear and those competing voices. Only the man himself can find the courage to be empathetic and reject violence and hate. How many men have such courage? Given the direction in which global society is heading, no doubt we will soon have an answer.

So much is yet to play for in the gender revolution, at least for men. In contrast, most women have already decided where they stand and it is not in the 1950s, which makes the future very challenging for these two types of men:

1. The male fundamentalist (e.g. misogynist)
2. The traditionally minded guy (e.g. chauvinist)

These two types of responders to the gender revolution remain the majority of men, especially in regions such as South America, Central America, the Caribbean, the Middle East, South Asia, Africa, Eastern Europe and South East Asia. Both types of men draw on traditional/toxic/hegemonic masculinity in order to present 'manliness' within their specific culture, even though how they enact it and personify it will differ from man to man. Every male fundamentalist is a direct threat to any woman, while a typical traditionally minded guy might yet be enabled to exit his toxic masculine cave[237] and join his female neighbour in helping create a better, safer, less

---

[237] See Whitehead, S. (2021) for elaboration of the 'toxic masculine cave'. Part 4: Caves and Crossroads.

hostile, more sustainable world; he might still be persuaded to listen to his compassionate, empathetic self.

While the male fundamentalist may appear a new threat to women, the fact is, he's been around a long time – forms of gender apartheid and men's total control over every aspect of women's lives have not suddenly emerged in the twenty-first century, though it should shock and anger every woman on the planet that so many men can behave this way towards them and attempt to justify it in the name of religion, fears of emasculation, or whatever excuse they offer. If it doesn't shock women, then it's difficult to see what would. How much women are prepared to tolerate is one question that gets raised here, the other being how many men will stand up and support them? The next two chapters provide some answers to those two questions along with pointers for the direction in which global society is now heading.

It will be interesting to see how women, and those men with progressive masculinity, react to the male fundamentalists in power in the White House from 2025 to 2029 and even possibly beyond that. Because we can expect the misogynistic men, the frightened men, all the insecure men around the world, to see the election of Donald Trump and the vocal anti-feminism of Putin, Xi Jinping, Musk and others like them, as clear signals to push back at women's rights, and those of LGBTQ+ people and return to some imagined maleist 'utopia' more reflective of the Middle Ages. These men will react to the threat to their masculinity and power in the way that men have done so down the ages – aggressively and violently. This is what they are, it is what they do. Expect nothing less. There will be attempts to reverse equal opportunities legislation and, as has already happened with abortion rights (e.g. the overturning of Roe v Wade), further limit women's control of their own bodies. Women's employment rights, maternity rights and educational opportunities could also be under threat. Certainly, the GOP will look to attack the university sector as it recognises this to have been a signal influence on the growth in liberal values in the USA over the past seven decades. They will also aim to exercise dictatorial control over compulsory education and reduce if not eliminate all DEIJ (Diversity, Equality, Inclusion and Justice) discourses and influences.

All very grim, though at least the male fundamentalists are no longer hiding behind weasel words. They are now very public.

The difficulty, if not serious challenge, facing heterosexual women is their sexuality: their biological need for men. It is like falling in love with the enemy. But even that hard statement doesn't cover the issue because clearly not all men are the enemy. How are women, especially young more vulnerable women, going to be able to differentiate between these types of men and their very contrasting masculinities? A significant number of men are extremely dangerous to all women, but especially those women who fall in love with them. Are women waking up to this reality? Possibly, certainly in those countries where men have become openly abusive towards all women and not caring to conceal their hatred of them – South Korea and the rise of the 4B movement is one example at time of writing. But male fundamentalism is not confined to a few countries – every country suffers from this problem to varying degrees, making every woman a potential victim.

The one standout question which each straight woman will have to ask herself is – which do I love more, men or independence? How women as a gender group answer that will determine the future of sex and the future of the genders. What we can see so far is that women's desire for independence from men is not going to disappear no matter how threatening men are to them. In the final reckoning, women are a whole lot stronger than men and have much more to lose by submitting to them. This is why this particular revolution, though a long time in the offing, is now unstoppable. The world has changed dramatically in less than a century and the speed of change is not lessening; if anything it is increasing. And central to this change, and the gender revolution, is knowledge combined with self-belief: this is the new independent femininity.

Men must accept and learn to live with this new gender arrangement because traditional male responses, including violence and misogyny, won't cut it any more:

> *'We cannot all succeed when half of us are held back. We call upon our sisters around the world to be brave – to embrace strength within themselves and realize their potential.'* Malala Yousafzai

> *'If not me, who? If not now, when?'* Emma Watson

> *'Of course I am not worried about intimidating men. The type of man who will be intimidated by me is exactly the type of man I have no interest in'.* Chimamanda Ngozi Adichie

> *'When they go low, we go high. That's not about hitting back, but keeping our souls intact when fighting for justice.'* Alexandria Ocasio-Cortez

Chapter 4: Men's Responses

'This movement is constantly being called a watershed moment. Even now, they're trying to see its demise. But it's not going anywhere.' Tarana Burke

'Women around the world are on the move, and a change is coming... a sense of movement has been unleashed and it will be very hard to stop it.' Helen Daouphars

'You cannot stop change. The younger generation know exactly what is out there. Everything's at our fingertips.' Raha Moharrak

'I think what we want to say to the women of Indonesia is, don't be afraid of being different. Don't be afraid to shout your independence.' Bracepot

'I don't pretend to be neutral. I think neutrality is dishonest. In fact, I think it's a disservice.' Nikole Hannah-Jones

'The most beautiful thing a woman can wear is confidence.' Huda Kattan

'Every woman's success should be an inspiration to another. We're strongest when we cheer each other on.' Serena Williams

'Your silence serves no one.' Danai Gurira.

Chapter 5: Living Apart, Growing Apart

Yorkshire is the largest and in my (biased) opinion, the most outstanding of all the English counties. If you've never been, just take a trip to Wharfedale and walk beside the gentle River Wharfe as it meanders alongside the picturesque ruins of a twelfth-century Augustinian monastery, long known as Bolton Abbey. And reflect not just on the peace and beauty but on the harshness behind it. For Yorkshire is a county with a troubled history; of strife, wars and poverty, where the working man had over the centuries lived in 'continual fear and danger of violent death', with life for him being 'solitary, poor, nasty, brutish and short.'[238]

And that was just the men of Yorkshire. How would Thomas Hobbes have described the lives of Yorkshire women?

Ambrose Whitehead was a typically gritty Yorkshireman. Born in 1794 he lived all his 83 years in one of the most unforgiving of environments, up on the windswept, starkly bleak Nidderdale moorland of Greenhow Hill; originally a Norse settlement and at 1,300 feet the highest village in Yorkshire. But long before the Vikings, there were the Romans. And it was they who discovered lead under those moors and mined them. Over 1,500 years later and lead was still being mined; not least by Ambrose.[239]

Ambrose started courting Elizabeth Bell from the nearby hamlet of Wath, in 1813. She was just fourteen. By then, Ambrose, aged nineteen, had already been a lead-miner for four years and it showed; not just his musculature, but in the grime that he could never fully scrub away. At least he had his four limbs – many miners lost theirs deep underground. Medical care was laudanum, leeches and the knife.

Ambrose and Elizabeth courted for two years and married in the summer of 1815, a few weeks after Wellington destroyed Napoleon's dreams of empire at the Battle of Waterloo. Elizabeth started giving birth at the age of sixteen. Twenty-five years later and she was still giving birth. Thomas Whitehead, her last child, was born in 1841. A quarter of a century of

---

[238] https://www.oxfordreference.com/display/10.1093/acref/9780191826719.001.0001/q-oro-ed4-00005474

[239] https://greenhow-hill.org.uk/

birthing; pregnant on average every fifteen months, with most pregnancies not going to term. Half her children died within the first three years. Seven survived to adulthood, one of whom was John Moss Whitehead, my great-great-grandfather. John Moss proved to be even more prolific than his father, siring twelve children between 1862 and 1879, nine of whom made it to adulthood.

All this reproduction, year after year, took place in a remote village on one of the highest moors of Yorkshire with no electricity, no medical care, no welfare state, no schooling, limited travel and little communication with the world beyond, but a lot of religion – Methodist, mostly. Tough on the men, but absolutely appalling for the women.

The Whiteheads of Greenhow Hill continued to 'enjoy' the processes of reproduction into the twentieth century. By the 1960s they were spreading around the world, though their breeding efforts had slowed by two-thirds to less than three children per family, which was typical of UK families of the time.

I was the eldest of three children. My sister, brother and I went on to have nine children between us.

Those nine children (currently aged between twenty-four and fifty) have so far produced *just two children* and that is solely thanks to my sister's daughter.

I am 75, and still no sign of being a grandfather. Not even much chance of attending a wedding. Of the nine great-great-great-great-great-grandkids of Ambrose, offspring of just one branch of the Whiteheads of Greenhow Hill, only three are married, and one of those is a common-law marriage. Needless to say, none of the family visits the Yorkshire Methodist churches any more.

My family's story of the past two hundred years is repeated around the world. Not identical in every detail, but very similar: steeply declining birth rates, declining marriage rates, rising divorce rate, rising number of singletons, solo lives, silo living, and a consequent growing separation of the sexes.

But that is not all of it. In the past twelve months, from conception of this book, new and unfamiliar changes between men and women have become noticeable – celibacy for example. And bisexuality. Topped off by a growing political divergence between liberal women and conservative men; a gender gap that some commentators describe as 'stark and staggering'.[240]

---

[240] https://www.nbcnews.com/politics/elections/young-men-women-are-taking-poll-gender-gap-staggering-new-levels-rcna202672

You could metaphorically drown in all the data, documents, articles and media comment fast being generated on these momentous changes to human society and repeated around the world in families like the Whiteheads of Yorkshire. Many thousands of experts, politicians, media folk and casual observers, each attempting to understand, interpret, explain and – in many cases predict – what all this means for the human race.

For me, it is all rather simple. Admittedly, maybe too simple, for I can encapsulate all these portentous changes in just one question to you.

Which life would you have rather had, Ambrose's or Elizabeth's?

The One?

Maybe Elizabeth Bell was in love with Ambrose when they married in the summer of 1815. Maybe she went to her wedding bed a virgin; excited, shy, expectant, demure and curious. Was she still in love with Ambrose twenty-five years and endless pregnancies later? Or had the bedroom, over those two-and-a-half decades, been transformed from Elizabeth's place of romantic sexual dreams into a place of pain, ordeal, disappointment, perhaps at times great frustration, and very bad dreams?

At least Ambrose had the Miner's Arms pub,[241] a few hundred yards walk from his tiny stone cottage, wherein he could submerge himself in beery manliness with his miner pals. One day in the not-too-distant future, his son, John Moss, would own that same pub and serve those same miners. But not their wives. Pregnant or not, women were excluded from this man's world.

Like women down the centuries, and even to this day, young Elizabeth would likely have yearned to find The One; the ideal man with whom she could settle down to married life, have children and raise her family.

The children, at least, she achieved, though it came at a high price: a quarter of a century of conception, pregnancy, birth and, tragically, miscarriage and infant death. Not fun. Not sexy. And certainly not romantic. But very commonplace for women throughout history.

But whether she was happy or miserable, Elizabeth had to carry on. Painful, emotionally and physically as it would unquestionably have been, she would have rationalised her situation, her predicament, in straightforward terms: this is the life that women have.

They have no choice.

---

[241] https://www.closedpubs.co.uk/yorkshire/greenhow_minersarms.html

Women Finally Getting to Choose

When women get to choose and feel empowered, interesting things happen. One of them is that long-held assumptions about femininity and female identity get swept away. For example, how many times I have been told about 'women's biological clock' I cannot recall, but it is many. And I believed it myself, which is part of the reason why I have five children; being anxious not to miss the clock's deadline with at least two of my wives. All I can say about the biological clock of women – their fertility window – is that nowadays it doesn't tick for very long. And it starts late. In the 1970s and even into the 1980s, the clock was still ticking loudest for women in their twenties. Today, women don't appear to hear it until their thirties – if they hear it at all.[242] Which is one reason why humanity is falling off a fertility cliff – and it won't be a soft landing for many countries, if they even survive as countries.

Birth Rates, Childlessness and Single Motherhood

It took the Whitehead family approximately one hundred years to see their fertility rate fall from more than six children per woman to fewer than three children per woman. A dramatic decline but slow compared to many other families around the world. In the USA, the same rate of decline took 82 years; Malaysia, 37 years; Thailand, 35 years; South Korea, eighteen years; China, eleven years; and Iran, ten years.[243] Many politicians assume this to be driven by the financial pressure on young couples. Well, billions of dollars in government incentives haven't reversed the 'alarming drop' in birth rates in South Korea, Japan or China.[244] Indeed, the situation is considered so

---

[242] The exception to this rule is African countries, especially sub-Saharan countries, where a high percentage (up to 70%) of women have their first birth before 20 years of age. https://equityhealthj.biomedcentral.com/articles/10.1186/s12939-020-01251-y#:~:text=Each%20year%2C%20an%20estimated%2016,%2Dincome%20countries%20%5B1%5D.

[243] https://ourworldindata.org/fertility-rate#:~:text=The%20global%20average%20was%20still,is%201.3%20children%20per%20woman

[244] In January 2025, Russia became the latest country offering financial incentives to encourage young women to have children. https://economictimes.indiatimes.com/news/international/global-trends/after-china-and-japan-now-russia-is-offering-100000-roubles-to-female-students-under-25-to-have-babies/articleshow/117076929.cms?from=mdr

desperate in China that government officials have taken to phoning women of childbearing age, asking 'are you pregnant yet?' and offering to remind them of 'the right time' to conceive a child.[245] But this is not just an Asian problem; it is worldwide. In 1950, the global fertility rate was still 4.84. At time of writing it is 2.23 (and that includes Africa where the rate is 4.20). By 2100 it will be down to 1.59. On that trend, some countries *will* disappear.[246]

In this book I am not attempting to decipher these demographics, because no one can pronounce a single explanation as to the many questions all this raises. I am concerned only with the consequences for gender relationships and the gender revolution. And they are starkly portended in comments such as these.[247]

> Heather: *'Done quite well flitting from job to job, country to country, free as a bird... at 55 still no f**ks given!'*

---

[245] https://www.independent.co.uk/asia/china/china-women-pregnancy-period-population-birth-rate-b2638734.html See also, https://www.voanews.com/a/7913276.html The Chinese government is now starting to ratchet up the pressure on young women to date, marry and give birth. If this 'soft' pressure does not produce results then I would forecast more draconian measures being applied. https://www.ft.com/content/5fdf42e1-2975-4c99-9031-a9f73c2251be

[246] https://ourworldindata.org/fertility-rate#:~:text=The%20global%20average%20was%20still,is%201.3%20children%20per%20woman https://geographical.co.uk/news/depopulation-the-major-countries-with-the-lowest-birth-rates-in-the-world https://www.euronews.com/health/2024/09/28/europes-fertility-crisis-which-european-country-is-having-the-fewest-babies https://www.newsweek.com/south-korea-news-population-faces-point-no-return-2005918

https://www.ndtv.com/feature/japan-will-disappear-5-points-on-countrys-population-crisis-3838478

But before countries disappear we can expect men to put severe pressure on women to have children. The signs of this are now becoming increasingly apparent in, for example, China, where women's 'loyalty and obedience' (to the state) is being aligned with a willingness to give birth. https://www.voanews.com/a/7913276.html A similar situation may emerge in Vietnam, another communist state facing dramatic demographic problems as one of the world's fastest aging countries . https://e.vnexpress.net/news/perspectives/aging-before-prosperity-vietnam-s-challenge-4829652.html#

[247] https://www.threads.net/@theofficialkatya/post/C9AZIGCttFp/women-in-their-50s-i-am-childless-and-have-no-regrets-about-it-the-comments-so-y

Rose: *'I'm 55, childfree by choice, and – shockingly – I do have a purpose in life! How weird! People who present female can do meaningful things other than pop out babies! Who knew'*

Anya: *'I'm 44 and decided pretty much as a teenage that I didn't want to have kids. One live birth video was enough to convince me, plus a host of other reasons. I briefly thought I'd changed my mind in my twenties, but by my mid thirties I was like "yeahhh no, definitely, no." I sing and travel for a living and absolutely love my life, I cannot imagine it another way.'*

Maggie: *'68, childless, never married, and NO REGRETS.'*

Joan: *'54, childless by choice and still thrilled about it. No regrets. Not for a moment.'*

Lisa: *'No regrets! I've had people ask me... do you hate children? Um??? And I think... geesh, these people still have no clue that they are asking questions to prove a point instead of actually want to know the answer!'*

What is striking is the enthusiasm these women, several over fifty, show for being childless. This is just a sample of such comments available on the web. I could fill the book with similar. As one of the above women wryly observes, *'who knew?'* Indeed.

Also now being tested to breaking-point concerns the role of men in the whole process of reproduction; e.g. how essential are they?, Following which, women's 'biological' maternalistic need for them. Admittedly, in this regard, men's role has never been that great. Aside from the act of penetration and insemination, most men through history and even to the modern day contribute a minimum. To illustrate, once pregnant, a modern independent woman has no further need of a man. He can be around or not, and most are not. Women will advise the mother-to-be through pregnancy; be the midwives at the actual birth; help nurse and care for the baby; provide nursery facilities for the young child; and then be the primary educators of that child at least through to secondary school. Importantly, most mothers will come to find that it is other women, not men, who provide the essential long-term emotional support as friends, family, colleagues, acquaintances and professionals.

By way of example, one British single woman friend of mine decided in her mid-thirties to have a baby. Being a full-time professional musician, she looked around for an equally gifted male musician, her reasoning being that two gifted musicians are likely to produce a third gifted musician. The man she chose lived in a van and jobbed from orchestra to orchestra as the work arose; a nomadic existence which suited his personality. There was never any question of my friend allowing this man into her life. She lived in a beautiful detached home, had lots of female friends, and was happily independent in every way. She put the 'arrangement' to the prospective father and he agreed to provide the necessary sperm through intercourse. Twenty years on, her son studies at music college while the 'father' intermittently flits in and out of his son's life as his lifestyle permits.

An example of men being used for what they can naturally provide, and nothing more. One way to look at this is as tables turned.

And then there are the growing number of women deciding they don't want a man to play any role whatsoever in their child's life. Not even the sex bit.[248]

Sophie starting hearing her biological clock ticking in her late thirties, having spent most of the previous decade living 'a really full, fun, happy life'. Her career in the RAF enabled her to fund the £30,000 it cost for IVF treatment. She now has a three-year old daughter.

Gina also got serious about being a mum in her mid-thirties. She got pregnant via IUI (intrauterine insemination) procedure using donor sperm. "If you're at a place where you want to have a child and you've got love and support around you, why wait for a man?" she said.

Michelle, 42, now has two children via IUI using sperm donors. "I had a long-term partner," she said, "but when that relationship ended I felt I didn't have time to find a man with whom to have a natural relationship. Having children is time-limited, finding a romantic partner is not."

Between 2012 and 2022, the number of single women in the UK having IVF or artificial insemination treatment more than tripled to just under 5,000; 6% of all IVF cycles are now in women without a partner.

> 'Ultimately, the choice to become a single mother through IUI or IVT is a manifestation of personal empowerment. Women are taking control of their reproductive destinies, embracing the challenges and joys of single motherhood with a sense of autonomy and determination.'[249]

---

[248] https://www.bbc.com/news/articles/c99relz9x4po

[249] https://newayfertility.com/blog/why-more-women-are-choosing-to-become-single-moms-with-iui-or-ivf/

Studies also show that increasing numbers of women are choosing to freeze their eggs in order to possibly have children later in life, and the main driver behind that decision is the partnership problems that women have with men, including the difficulty of 'finding suitable partners'.[250]

> 'The lack of suitable partners rather than career or educational ambitions, is why more women are trying to prolong their fertility. This 'men as partners problem' is usually talked about for men in the global south, now we need to start talking about the men as partners problem for women in the global north.'[251]

Childlessness, single motherhood, artificial insemination, egg freezing – each is a manifestation of women making massive lifestyle choices without the involvement of men, without being held accountable to men. And then there is marriage and divorce.

Marriage, Divorce and Cohabitation

Since the 1970s, divorce has become more popular than marriage, at least in the West. In the US, marriage rates have fallen by nearly 60% in the past fifty years, while globally they are at their lowest point in recorded history.[252] Men born in my year, 1949, had an 80% likelihood of being married by the age of twenty-five. British men born thirty years later had just a 10% likelihood of walking down the aisle with their beloved by the same age.[253]

The 1970s, the decade when radical feminism impacted on global society, was also a significant decade for divorce; 48% of American couples who married in the 1970s were divorced within twenty-five years. In the

---

[250] https://www.cnbc.com/2024/03/30/a-look-at-why-many-women-undergo-egg-freezing-and-the-costs-associated-with-it.html

[251] https://www.theguardian.com/society/2023/apr/23/motherhood-women-freeze-eggs-male-partners-men-fertility See also, Inhorn. M.C. (2023) *Motherhood On Ice. The mating gap and why women freeze their eggs.* New York: NYU Press.

[252] https://spectrumnews1.com/oh/columbus/news/2023/03/10/u-s--marriage-rate-plummets-nearly-60--over-the-past-50-years--study-reveals https://onlinemftprograms.com/worldwide-marriage-statistics/#:~:text=Globally%2C%20marriage%20rates%20have%20been,lowest%20point%20in%20recorded%20history.

[253] https://ourworldindata.org/marriages-and-divorces

UK, Norway, Sweden, Austria, Canada and South Korea, divorce rates more than tripled between 1970 and the millennium. Countries which have seen a significant rise in divorce rates (more than doubling) since 2000 include Ireland, Mexico, Turkey, Singapore, Russia, Greece, Thailand, Poland, Japan, Spain, Brazil, China and Iran.[254] By way of example, in the first three months of 2025, China saw an 8% drop in marriage registrations with a simultaneous 10% increase in divorce registrations compared to the same period of 2024.[255]

The USA and Canada are arguably now the world's first unofficial 'post-marriage societies', with less than 50% of adults aged eighteen or over being married.[256] The population of Canada in 2021 was 38.23 million, of which only 37.75% were married.[257] The USA also has one of the highest divorce rates for first marriages – 45%, rising to 60% for second marriages, and 73% for third marriages.[258] Far from being 'happy ever after', the average first marriage now lasts just eight years. That's in the USA. In France it is just five years.[259] This is not marriage so much as serial monogamy accredited in law.

While the last twenty-five years has seen a marginal slowing down of the divorce rate in some countries, this appears due to couples waiting longer before getting married. For example, the average age of men marrying

---

[254] Ibid

[255] https://www.bangkokpost.com/world/3013121/more-chinese-leave-the-knot-untied-as-marriage-registrations-drop

[256] https://medium.com/@yye7/what-would-a-post-marriage-society-look-like-470da502610a

[257] https://nussbaumlaw.ca/marriage-statistics-in-canada/

[258] https://ourworldindata.org/marriages-and-divorces#:~:text=For%20those%20married%20in%20the,were%20divorced%20within%2025%20years. https://www.nytimes.com/2021/10/20/opinion/marriage-decline-america.html https://www.marketwatch.com/story/fewer-than-50-of-u-s-adults-are-now-married-its-time-to-give-more-legal-and-financial-breaks-to-single-people-law-professor-says-11664992681 https://www150.statcan.gc.ca/n1/daily-quotidien/220713/dq220713b-eng.htm https://www.usatoday.com/story/life/health-wellness/2024/09/05/marriage-divorce-rate/74899214007/

[259] https://www.verywellmind.com/how-many-marriages-end-in-divorce-facts-and-figures-7487050

women in the UK rose from 27 in 1972 to just under forty by 2019, with women's average age being 25 and 37 respectively.[260]

Looking at global statistics on marriage and divorce can be akin to walking into a maze with numerous entrances but only one exit, not least because while there are distinctive trends, there are significant differences between countries and between cultures. For example, divorce is still illegal in the Philippines (for Roman Catholics), while India has historically had a low divorce rate (1%) – not because all married couples are happy but because divorce has been a taboo subject, leading to mental abuse, neglect, physical abuse and long-term permanent separations. However, that taboo is quickly lessening and at least in the urban Indian population divorce is now on a steep curve upwards.[261]

Across the Muslim world, e.g. Saudi Arabia, it is incredibly difficult for women to instigate divorce, with husbands having 'unilateral repudiation', able to exercise power and control over the whole process, including forcing their wives to give up all their financial rights and property entitlements.[262] However, following years of protest by women, the controversial triple talaq, the traditional and quick way for Muslim men to get divorced, was recently banned in many Muslim countries or countries with a large Muslim population, including India, Saudi Arabia, UAE, Pakistan, Bangladesh, Morocco and Malaysia.[263] Though in non-Muslim countries such as the UK, which permit informal (without legal authority) Sharia councils/courts and consequently have a large number of Islamic marriages, Muslim women can still find themselves culturally and socially trapped in abusive relationships.[264]

---

[260] https://time.com/5434949/divorce-rate-children-marriage-benefits/   https://journals.sagepub.com/doi/10.1177/2378023119873497

[261] https://www.linkedin.com/pulse/why-divorce-increasing-2024-fastrack-legal-solutions-zf4mc#:~:text=Infidelity%20and%20Trust%20Issues&text=However%2C%20with%20the%20advent%20of,contributing%20to%20higher%20divorce%20rates.   https://adjuvalegal.com/divorce/divorce-rate-in-india/#:~:text=The%20rate%20of%20divorce%20in,increased%20divorce%20rate%20in%20India.

[262] https://www.hrw.org/news/2023/03/08/saudi-arabia-law-enshrines-male-guardianship

[263] https://www.bbc.com/news/world-asia-india-49160818

[264] https://rlplawgroup.com/places-around-the-world-with-difficult-divorce-laws   https://www.netlawman.co.in/ia/talaq

What has unquestionably increased in popularity is cohabitation. From being unacceptable when I was a teenager, cohabitation has become normalised around the world. The UK is a prime example. In England and Wales, the total number of cohabiting couples increased by 144% between 1996 and 2021. Across Scandinavia and in countries such as Germany, Canada and France, cohabitation is now more common than marriage. Indeed, there are few if any countries where cohabitation is on the decline.[265]

The gender mostly driving all these changes is not men, but women.

- 70% of divorces are instigated by women.[266]
- Women are less likely to want to get married than men.[267]
- Women are more reluctant to cohabit unless they are in love, while men's main reason for cohabitation is sex.[268]
- Women are less likely to be seeking romance than men.[269]
- Women are now seeking partners who align with their education and career ambitions.[270]

---

[265] https://population-europe.eu/research/popdigests/living-together-without-getting-married#:~:text=In%20Norway%20and%20France%2C%20more,only%20in%20Sweden%20and%20Estonia. https://www.stewartslaw.com/news/the-state-of-cohabitation-law-in-the-uk/#:~:text=The%20rise%20of%20cohabitation%20in%20the%20UK&text=It%20is%2C%20therefore%2C%20perhaps%20unsurprising,around%203.6%20million%20in%202021. https://www.psychologytoday.com/us/blog/happy-singlehood/202201/cohabitation-is-rising-globally#:~:text=Fears%20of%20commitment%20to%20marriage,all%20%5B1%2D3%5D.

[266] https://affinitypsych.com/why-do-women-initiate-divorce-more-frequently-than-men/#:~:text=You%20may%20or%20may%20not,number%20is%20only%2027%20percent.

[267] https://uh.edu/news-events/stories/2023/january-2023/011123.php https://www.pewresearch.org/social-trends/2014/09/24/chapter-1-public-views-on-marriage/

[268] https://news.umich.edu/he-says-she-says-men-and-women-view-living-together-very-differently/

[269] https://www.newsnationnow.com/us-news/more-women-choose-single-married/

[270] ibid

Trying to get a clear picture of how young people see marriage isn't easy because there are conflicting data. An overwhelming majority of American Gen Z respondents claim to be open to the possibility of getting married, with one in two saying they 'definitely' see it happening.[271] However, this is in conflict with the reality, which is that Gen Z are dating less than any previous generation, *with 44% of men reporting having no relationship experience during their teen years,* double the rate for older men.[272] This fits with 2022 US Census Bureau statistics confirming that more than one in three (34%) people fifteen years and older have never been married. That's up from one in four in 1950.[273] A telling statistic is that 41% of men and a staggering 52% of women think marriage is an outdated tradition.[274] And the main reason women aren't planning to wed? Apparently, it is because they are just not interested in the arrangement.

Regardless of religious beliefs, marriage is going out of fashion, becoming an outdated concept across all age groups and has been doing so at least since the 1970s, not just in the West but globally. Apart from countries with powerful patriarchies (e.g. Saudi Arabia) and/or intransigent traditional cultures, divorce is no longer taboo and has risen dramatically since the 1950s. Cohabitation is fast replacing marriage, though such relationships are generally seen as less committed and more likely to be temporary, e.g. typically twenty-four months. Both sexes see cohabitation as an expected part of life, but also less of a commitment than marriage, and therefore less of a limitation on their freedom.

If the Whitehead's of Greenhow Hill suddenly landed back on earth after been frozen in time for the past hundred years, what would they make of all this? No doubt they'd be appalled. Well, certainly the men might be. Perhaps the women would start celebrating.

---

[271] https://www.theknotww.com/press-releases/10205/#:~:text=Eighty%2Done%20percent%20of%20Gen,the%20average%20age%20being%2028.

[272] https://www.americansurveycenter.org/commentary/gen-zs-romance-gap-why-nearly-half-of-young-men-arent-dating/

[273] https://www.census.gov/newsroom/press-releases/2022/americas-families-and-living-arrangements.html#:~:text=Marriage:,at%2Dhome%20father%20in%202022.

[274] https://thrivingcenterofpsych.com/blog/millennials-gen-z-marriage-expectations-statistics/

Women's desire or need for The One may not be quite as strong as it was in Elizabeth Bell's day, but then nor are the reasons for women to get married. Women have more options and given the chance, they will most definitely exercise them. This is independent femininity in action. Men, on the other hand, still hold on to the idea of marriage as a route into manhood and regular sex, but are finding it increasingly difficult to find women who value marriage as much as they do. For one thing, women cannot see what benefits it will bring them, while men can. Men also tend to fall in love more easily than do women, and it is women who are more likely to end a relationship, and certainly more likely to anticipate the breakup.[275]

Cohabitation becomes one way through this maze – a softer option for both sexes, enabling them to experiment with sexual commitment without holding them down to any legal promises, contractual obligations or a long-term fate such as was the lot of Elizabeth and her female peers back in the 'good ol days'.

This all suggests that women, while traditionally being seen as the romantic, emotionally vulnerable gender, easily deluded into love and marriage, are a lot more hard-headed and relationship-savvy than most men.

Solo, Silo, Lifestyles

Despite the hard life they had, I doubt my ancestors of Greenhow Hill were ever lonely. How could they be with all those kids, grandkids, nephews and nieces, aunties and uncles, packed into neat rows of Yorkshire stone cottages up on the desolate moors? They had family around them day and night, like them or not. It is all rather different nowadays.

In August 2024, a report came out of Japan stating that 40,000 Japanese died alone in their homes during the first half of the year.[276] What was remarkable was that the Japanese ever noticed. After all, this is a country that even has a word for 'all the lonely people'; ohitorisama, which translates as being single and not caring about, or for, anyone else. That is silo living,

---

[275] https://www.vice.com/en/article/why-men-fall-in-love-faster-than-women/#:~:text=And%20while%20societal%20and%20cultural,and%20meaningful%2C%20loving%20relationships.%E2%80%9D https://www.psychologytoday.com/intl/blog/it-s-man-s-and-woman-s-world/201502/who-is-more-likely-leave-bad-relationship#:~:text=Women%20also%20tend%20to%20be,emotional%20support%20(McClintock%202014).

[276] https://www.bbc.com/news/articles/cwyx6wwp5d5o

not just solo living.[277] And there are a lot of Japanese living like this; 34% of all households, some eighteen million, are single person households. While these singles may live alone, the truth is they have a lot of company. In China, the singles population was expected to reach a record 400 million in 2024, doubling since 2018. More than half of Chinese aged 25–29 are now living solo lives, many living silo lives.[278] The percentage of singles is even greater in South Korea, which now has 42% of all households as single-person.[279] If you imagine this to be a uniquely Asian phenomena then you'd be mistaken. In the USA, 46.4% of the adult population are single, up from just 22% in 1950.[280] The UK has seen singletons rise to 30% of all households, 8.4 million people, with the number of women not living in a couple or who have never married, rising in every age range under seventy.[281] Even countries with a traditionally strong marriage culture, such as Thailand, Saudi Arabia, Vietnam, Nigeria, India and Pakistan are seeing a rise in singletons.[282] It is an unstoppable trend, cutting across class, religious, racial and ethnic lines. Globally, there are now over two billion single people – a quarter of the world's population and about a third of

---

[277] Solo living is living alone but possibly with a romantic partner. Silo living is living a largely isolated existence with no close relationships.

[278] https://www.aninews.in/news/world/asia/chinas-single-population-to-reach-400-million-youths-staring-at-being-single-for-life20230223234719/#:~:text=China's%20single%20population%20to%20reach,Representative%20Image https://www.voanews.com/a/china-faces-record-high-unmarried-rate-among-young-people/7426303.html

[279] https://www.koreaherald.com/article/3295607

[280] https://www.statista.com/statistics/242022/number-of-single-person-households-in-the-us/#:~:text=In%202023%2C%20approximately%2038.1%20million,households%20in%20the%20United%20States.

[281] https://www.ons.gov.uk/peoplepopulationandcommunity/birthsdeathsandmarriages/families/bulletins/familiesandhouseholds/2023#:~:text=4.,number%20of%20people%20living%20alone.

[282] https://www.statista.com/topics/999/singles/#editorsPicks https://www.euromonitor.com/article/half-the-worlds-new-single-person-households-to-emerge-in-asia-pacific https://wearesololiving.com/countries-solo-households-commonplace/ https://www.weforum.org/stories/2020/01/living-alone/ https://iusw.org/how-many-people-are-single-in-the-world/

all people over fifteen years of age.[283],[284] Ohitorisama has become a global phenomenon – the 'super solo' society is now well and truly with us.[285]

But there is also a significant gender gap in these statistics. Not surprisingly, due to China's imbalanced gender ratio, around 55% of men and 39% of women are single.[286] But a similar gender gap in singletons is apparent around the world: Vietnam, USA, the UK, Brazil, South Africa, Japan, Singapore, India and Canada are just a few of the countries where single men outnumber single women.[287] A 2019 study predicted that by 2030, 45% of women between the ages of 25–44 will be childless and single. A contentious (2023) Pew Research report, suggested the US is now on the way to that scenario if not already reached it; among young adults, one third of women and 'an astonishing 63% of men' are single – a thirty-point gender gap.[288]

> 'Men in their twenties are more likely than women in their twenties to be romantically uninvolved, sexually dormant, friendless and lonely. They stand at the vanguard of an epidemic of declining marriage, sexuality and relationships that afflicts all of young America... This is a crisis of connection.'[289]

---

[283] https://iusw.org/how-many-people-are-single-in-the-world/

[284] https://medium.com/the-savanna-post/apparently-1-in-4-adults-will-stay-single-for-their-whole-life-but-is-this-actually-true-f8758be01ae9#:~:text=Research%20has%20circulated%20recently%20that,will%20stay%20single%20for%20life.

[285] https://www.bbc.com/worklife/article/20200113-the-rise-of-japans-super-solo-culture

[286] https://www.statista.com/statistics/1258197/china-share-of-singles-by-gender/

[287] https://www.bloomberg.com/news/articles/2015-02-11/where-there-are-more-single-men-than-women https://www.vice.com/en/article/these-countries-now-have-a-historic-imbalance-of-men-to-women/

[288] https://ifstudies.org/blog/number-3-in-2023-theres-no-huge-gender-gap-in-being-single-among-young-adults. The top five US cities with the 'most skewed' gender gap, ratio of unmarried men to unmarried women were, in 2023, San Jose, Austin, Colorado Springs, Seattle, and Mesa, Arizona, with typically 120+ men for every 100 women. https://www.seattletimes.com/seattle-news/data/seattle-has-one-of-the-highest-ratios-of-single-men-to-single-women/

[289] https://thehill.com/blogs/blog-briefing-room/3868557-most-young-men-are-single-most-young-women-are-not/ https://www.reddit.com/r/Futurology/

Perhaps, but not a crisis of connection for young women so much as for young men. For women, this is singlehood not as a 'failure' to avoid spinsterhood or fear of being labelled a 'left-over woman' but singlehood via agency, empowerment and choice. All the drivers behind the rise in independent femininity explored in previous chapters – education, economics, career, globalisation – configure to create the circumstances by which women can say 'no' to marriage, say 'maybe' to cohabitation, and say 'very unlikely' to parenting – if they choose to.[290]

Do women feel they are 'missing out' by being single? It would appear not, despite the continual strength of the 'coupledom narrative' in modern society.[291] As one researcher put it:

> *'When I published my research claiming that single women without children were happier than married ones, I was taken aback by the response. I had lots of emails from single women saying thank you, because people might start believing them when they say they are actually doing all right. There are competing narratives for women, so some will be challenged internally because their experiences (of being single) are more positive than society expects them to be.'*[292]

> *'Women take to single life more readily than men. On every question that was asked in the study, single women were more comfortable than single men with their single lives. They were less likely to want a romantic partner. They were more sexually satisfied.'*[293]

That single women would be happier than married women should not surprise us. After all, and as I discuss below, marriage can be a trap for women, often leading to mental and physical abuse, a diminishment of self-

---

comments/1195kb7/us_most_young_men_are_single_most_young_women_are/?t

[290] https://www.reddit.com/r/science/comments/1gimp2p/women_take_to_single_life_more_readily_than_men/?rdt=52301

[291] https://www.theguardian.com/lifeandstyle/2021/jan/17/why-are-increasing-numbers-of-women-choosing-to-be-single

[292] https://www.theguardian.com/lifeandstyle/2021/jan/17/why-are-increasing-numbers-of-women-choosing-to-be-single https://journals.sagepub.com/doi/10.1177/19485506241287960

[293] https://www.reddit.com/r/science/comments/1gimp2p/women_take_to_single_life_more_readily_than_men/?rdt=52301

esteem, depression and mental health problems, especially for those women who have absorbed hegemonic/traditional femininity. Today's women are well aware of the risks to them personally that come with marriage – at least they should be, because there is no shortage of evidence. Women who are single have largely chosen to be. Men, on the other hand, prefer not to be alone. They don't choose a singleton lifestyle, they invariably have it forced upon them due to not being able to find a partner, the incels being a prime example. This problem is compounded for men, especially those with traditional masculinity; they are less skilled at creating positive human relationships and long-lasting friendships, and are more likely to rely on a romantic partner for emotional support. This makes being single a trap for men, a threat to their mental health and wellbeing. The opposite applies for women; they are much more likely to enjoy being single – they don't need men to avoid loneliness.[294]

> Lusi: 'Women have more friends than men do. When men are not in a relationship they're more lonely, when women are not in a relationship they still have friends.'
>
> Mandi: 'Historically, women didn't necessarily want relationships with men, they needed them to survive. This is no longer the case.'
>
> Cath: 'Most single women are that way by choice whereas most single men would prefer not to be alone. It's a lot harder to be happy single when you don't want to be.'
>
> Joan: 'The single biggest mistake a woman can make in terms of happiness is marrying a man. It's been shown time and time again.'

All of which raises many questions, a key one being how do young men feel about this? Here are some revealing quotes taken from www.reddit.com.[295]

> McDunky: 'Everyone says "all you need is love" but many of us 20+ young adult men have been running on empty our entire lives.'

---

[294] https://www.americansurveycenter.org/why-mens-social-circles-are-shrinking/?t

[295] https://www.reddit.com/r/Futurology/comments/1195kb7/us_most_young_men_are_single_most_young_women_are/?t   https://www.reddit.com/r/science/comments/1gimp2p/women_take_to_single_life_more_readily_than_men/?rdt=52301

Chapter 5: Living Apart, Growing Apart

Mammoth: *'I'm a happy man living on the fringes of society. I don't really like any other people but I'm not some dangerous lunatic. I've lived like this since I left uni 20+ years ago. I don't really engage in society in any noticeable way.'*

Kaowser: *'I'm a 35 yr old male. Struggling with finding love. Not matched on eharmony yet. Should I just give up?'*

Iguess06: *'I'm 34. I'm done trying and caring. If something comes along I'm open to it. But I don't care to waste more time worrying about these things. It is what it is.'*

Utastelikebacon: *'I'm a single man in my thirties and I have never felt more distant from the opposite sex in my life. Honestly I don't know what is going on.'*

Anon: *'My teenage son tells me all the girls at his school are lesbians.'*

Dallen13:*'"This is how radical men are made. Unless we are able to adapt. This will get worse.'*

Anon: *'As our society works through this, I think people are going to be shocked at the level of misandry we tolerate. We are setting young men up to fail at every level.'*

Batsniper: *'I'm a 26 yr old male. I go to work, come home, play with my dog, watch tv, and go to bed. The other week I recorded how many conversations I had and it was eight, six of which were coworkers. I've tried going out. I've gone to events, clubs, bars, dating apps. No one wants me around. I've accepted it. I long for a loving relationship or even a friend, but now I am just waiting to die alone.'*

The sadness is these comments is revealing – and worrying. How can we not feel compassion and empathy for young men such as these, suffering loneliness and isolation? Inadequate many may be, but they are a product of society. Lots of these men are not just living solo lives, they are living silo lives – socially isolated, largely removed from society. How many men are in this situation around the world? No one knows, but it must be many millions. Women are indeed 'doing it for themselves' and the wake-up call to men could not be louder, because whether they realise it or not, they are now in the midst of a growing 'relationship recession'.[296]

---

[296] One demographic adding to this problem is when a society has a surplus of males; usually arising in those cultures which have long favoured male children

> *'The trend is global. From the US, Finland and South Korea to Turkey, Tunisia and Thailand, falling birth rates are increasingly downstream of a relationship recession among young adults. Baby bonuses put the cart before the horse when a growing share of people are without a partner... The wider data on loneliness and dating frustrations suggests all is not well.'*[297]

Over the years I have encountered many single women, expert at 'doing it for themselves' especially in South East Asia; never married and childless by choice; professionals with careers. Three I met in Taiwan, each one unique but together representative of the new solo society in Asia. One is a thirty-something news presenter on national television who went on to do a PhD and pursue a part-time career in academia. The second is an American-Chinese woman, also in her thirties, with a doctorate in optometry from a US university; she was spending most of her thirties just travelling the world before returning to live with her family in Boston. The third is a Taiwanese academic and feminist, in her forties, briefly married and divorced in her twenties and single ever since. Aside from their level of education, these women are articulate, confident, with stable lives and good mental and physical wellbeing. They each exhibited independent femininity. Not that they didn't need men for sex at certain times; each woman pursued casual relationships or longer-term relationships as it suited them. But they retained total control over their lives. Men were ancillary – the support act in their life journey, not the directors of it, nor the reason for it. These single women are not in crisis. They are living life to the full.

In my lifetime, women around the world have gone from needing marriage in order to survive and prosper, having children in order to validate their traditional femininity and relying on men to provide for them, to almost total rejection of all those narratives and expectations. It is both extraordinary and revolutionary.

---

over females. In China and India the problem is especially acute with a projected 12-15% excess of young men over the next 20 years in both countries. Many of these men, often rural peasants, will remain single all their lives, never having a family or indeed a relationship with a woman. Such an imbalance could lead to increased anti-social behaviour, misogyny, crime and terrorism, and a general destabalisation of society. See: https://www.sciencedaily.com/releases/2006/08/060828211841.htm?t

[297] John Burn-Murdoch, (2025) https://www.ft.com/content/43e2b4f6-5ab7-4c47-b9fd-d611c36dad74

Celibacy

The anxiety, fear and insecurity that pervades traditional masculinity and men's sense of manliness comes in many forms but perhaps the most potent – yet most concealed and unacknowledged – concerns women's sexuality. How many men will admit to being intimidated by the sexual energy of women? How many men secretly compare their own sexual performance, invariably time-limited and exhausting, with that of their female partner – which is not time-limited and not exhausting but equally (if not more) satisfying? Every straight man, without exception. And why not? The whole edifice of hegemonic/toxic/traditional masculinity is built on compulsory heterosexuality and there's not much advantage in that unless as a man you can claim potency, high libido and all the myths of unbridled sexual performance as a thrusting, ever-hard, penis-defined, 'always up for it' male.

The fear that men have of women's sexuality (and of their own impotence when confronted with it) is such that throughout history they've gone to great lengths to hide it, to control it and to lessen it: covering women in black from head to toe; being unable to even gaze on a menstruating woman never mind have sex with her; burning widows; legislating against women having more than one husband; punishing women for adultery; creating the 'Madonna and whore' complex; obsessing over virginal females; denying even the existence of lesbians; and of course, rape and FGM – the ultimate male sanctions against women's sexuality and femininity.

All these actions, each designed to diminish women's sexuality and elevate that of men, merely confirm the obvious, which is that women have a stronger sex urge than men and men know it. This makes the rise in celibacy and sexless relationships one of the more powerful signals that women and men are pulling apart, leaving a lot of men marooned on their tiny island of male sexual mythology.

The rise of voluntary celibates has been evident in Japan and South Korea for over a decade but now we are seeing sexlessness go worldwide.[298]

In January 2024, Google reported a 90% increase in searches for celibacy in the UK, while by the middle of 2024, the #celibacy hashtag on TikTok had had more than 195m views, with many voluntary celibates claiming it improves their mental health and sense of wellbeing.[299] In the US, voluntary

---

[298] https://globalist.yale.edu/in-the-magazine/features/single-and-sexless-celibacy-syndrome-in-japan/

[299] https://www.vogue.com.au/beauty/hands-off-on-celibacy-voluntary-abstinence-or-going-sex-sober/news-story/7eff17ca1c9fddb13c94fa7a373eb774

celibacy has been on the rise for several years.[300] In 2021, the General Social Survey found that 25% of Americans over the age of eighteen hadn't had sex once in the previous twelve months – a thirty-year high.[301] Identical shifts in sexual behaviour are apparent around the world including in China, New Zealand, Australia, Canada, Belgium, Austria, Hong Kong and even that most romantic of countries, France.[302] And a constant key point in all these studies is that 'women find celibacy to be more satisfying than men do.'[303]

Admittedly, the research pointing to a rise in global celibacy remains unclear as to whether it is a temporary 'moment'[304] or something longer-lasting, but what is without question is that Gen Zs and Millennials especially are having less sex than any previous generation: 15% of young adults aged 20–24 born in the 1990s reported having had no sex partners since the age of eighteen, and are twice as likely to be virgins that GenXs, those born in the 1960s and 1970s.[305]

---

[300] https://www.huffingtonpost.co.uk/entry/celibacy-is-on-the-rise-should-you-consider-trying-it_uk_63d25bc3e4b0c2b49ada9810

[301] https://time.com/6978361/celibate-women-shaming-essay/

[302] https://www.rnz.co.nz/news/national/517325/why-young-people-are-turning-to-celibacy https://www.irishexaminer.com/lifestyle/people/arid-41450470.html https://www.independent.co.uk/life-style/love-sex/celibacy-bumble-julia-fox-sofie-hagen-b2545661.html https://www.sixthtone.com/news/1010510 https://www.spectator.co.uk/article/the-bizarre-sexual-politics-of-the-french/ https://www.theguardian.com/lifeandstyle/2023/apr/26/the-rise-of-voluntary-celibacy-most-of-the-sex-ive-had-i-wish-i-hadnt-bothered It is not just young women who are choosing voluntary celibacy, there is evidence of young men also rejecting physical intimacy with women: https://www.artefactmagazine.com/2023/05/25/male-volcels-why-are-more-young-men-choosing-voluntary-celibacy/ https://www.youtube.com/watch?v=flLn9n5Aalk, See also, Sherman, C. (2025) *The Second Coming and the Next Generation's Fight Over Its Future.* London: Gallery Books.

[303] https://inquiretalk.com/12-reasons-behind-trend-of-voluntary-celibacy/ https://www.elle.com/uk/life-and-culture/culture/a43156895/welcome-to-the-rise-of-celibacy/

[304] https://www.psychologytoday.com/intl/blog/the-myths-of-sex/202407/is-voluntary-celibacy-on-the-rise

[305] https://time.com/4435058/millennials-virgins-sex/ https://pmc.ncbi.nlm.nih.gov/articles/PMC7293001/#:~:text=This%20survey%20study%20found%20

What is also unclear is why it is happening. Certainly, it is a shift in societal attitudes and 'changing norms' but how much of this is a direct consequence of the rise in independent femininity remains to be seen. In other words, are women declaring a ban on sex with men, either consciously or subconsciously? That there is a growing movement amongst women for such a ban is evidenced in the 'radical feminist' 4B movement which originated in South Korea in 2019 and has since gone global, especially impacting in the USA following the 2024 Presidential election.[306] The 4Bs represent No sex with men, No giving birth, No dating men, No marriage with men. A more explicit rejection of men by women would be hard to find.[307]

But this growing disinterest in traditional romance is even impacting teenagers – a demographic not known for being uninterested in sex. At time of writing, a survey of Japanese high-school students found that 'an astonishing' four out of five teen boys had yet to experience their first kiss with a girl. Japanese girls have 'also become more chaste' with only 27.5% admitting to having had a first kiss, down from over 40% six years previously.[308] This reluctance to 'hook up' is supported by numerous Japanese surveys over the past decade, typically finding that a 'quarter of Japanese adults under forty are virgins, with the number increasing'.[309] In the

---

that,have%20implications%20for%20public%20health

[306] https://apple.news/A9C5HWH2dTXKx4GYHN3plkg   https://apple.news/Ap3VyRv-3QjuDCYW5ntrj5A   https://www.prestigeonline.com/my/lifestyle/culture-plus-entertainment/south-korean-4b-feminist-movement/

[307] https://www.theguardian.com/commentisfree/article/2024/may/21/celibacy-hetrosexual-women-boysober-4b-sex-positive-feminism   https://www.theguardian.com/world/2024/nov/15/4b-south-korea-feminist-movement-donald-trump-election-backlash?CMP=Share_iOSApp_Other   https://www.theguardian.com/us-news/2024/nov/07/4b-movement-trump-women?CMP=Share_iOSApp_Other

[308] https://www.scmp.com/week-asia/lifestyle-culture/article/3287792/japanese-teens-first-kiss-rate-drops-amid-disinterest-romance-sparking-demographic-fears?share=TTu%2BkkZuumK9ZLqsXzKAjQ8FSh3sul%2BK8q9C1zzdnD9gAFmXqTrZWgo%2FTLGcr%2F35x8szs%2ByKqAVeGx%2Bult%2FVQSPUBZrpYKtlE6zFIRWD8Qc%3D&utm_campaign=social_share

[309] https://globalist.yale.edu/in-the-magazine/features/single-and-sexless-celibacy-syndrome-in-japan/   https://www.forbes.com/sites/

UK, one in eight 26-year-olds are still virgins,[310] something unimaginable back when I was in my twenties; indeed, as I related in Chapter 3, most of my peers were married before they reached twenty-five.

Much of the research fails to distinguish between the involuntary celibacy of the men (e.g. incels) and the rise in voluntary celibacy across the genders, though whether voluntary or not, celibacy completely contradicts and undermines long-held notions about male sexual primacy which affirms it to be an 'overpowering instinct and barely controllable'.[311]

However, celibacy is just one part of this complex emerging mosaic of twenty-first century human sexuality. The other aspect is sexlessness in relationships, with 'heterosexual marriages experiencing high rates of sexlessness (25–50%).[312] One American psychologist puts this down to 'the battle of the sexes', though in China, where there are now identical trends,[313] the government is trying to avoiding the 'gender conflict' scenario and instead opting for more 'love education'.

> 'Colleges and universities should assume responsibility of providing marriage and love education to college students by offering marriage and love education courses. These measures would help create a healthy and positive marriage and childbearing cultural atmosphere.'[314]

If there is going to be hard evidence of women and men not just living apart but growing apart, one would expect to find it in human sexuality, not least because it is a biological impulse as much, if not more so, than a

---

ericmack/2019/04/07/a-quarter-of-japanese-adults-under-40-are-virgins-and-the-number-is-increasing/#:~:text=For%20women%20between%20the%20ages,older%20half%20of%20the%20cohort.

[310] https://www.dailymail.co.uk/news/article-5696417/Virgin-numbers-rise-UK-fear-intimacy.html

[311] Whitehead, S.M. (2002) P. 162. See Chapter 5, for discussion.

[312] https://www.psychologytoday.com/intl/blog/the-state-of-our-unions/202210/the-battle-of-the-sexes-has-left-more-couples-sexless

[313] https://www.researchgate.net/publication/26333719_Sexlessness_among_Married_Chinese_Adults_in_Hong_Kong_Prevalence_and_Associated_Factors https://journals.sagepub.com/doi/full/10.1177/2057150X221114599

[314] https://www.reuters.com/world/china/china-calls-universities-provide-love-education-2024-12-04/

sociological one. And evidence there is, with at least one sexologist is now declaring this to be a global phenomenon:

> 'There is a long-term trend among people, today, in general, for having less sex with few partners. Humans are increasingly less sexually active, with some foregoing sex altogether.'[315]

Women's Same-Sex Relationships

One of the advantages of being a woman with independent femininity is that you can have sex with whomever you like; young, old, male or female. Your gender identity construct does not act as an inhibitor and being an independent woman, you are not allowing traditional sexual values to inhibit you either. It is all a matter of choice.

It is totally the opposite for most straight men, trapped as they are in traditional/hegemonic/toxic masculinity. For these guys, sex with another male, unless performed as an act of rape, violence and expression of masculine power, is a definite no-no. Certainly, there can be no physical expression of love between such men. Even a bro-hug is limited to the sports arena or a drunken night out on the town for most guys; sadly also, for many fathers and sons. And a kiss on the lips between traditionally minded men remains totally taboo.

Women, on the other hand, are increasingly finding fun, if not a lot of pleasure, in kissing each other on the lips and elsewhere. Not just lesbians, who have been at this game for millennia, but straight women.

> 'In 2019, 65% of women reported only being attracted to men, a notable decrease from 77% in 2011. Surveys from around the world report the same trend. In that sense, eschewing exclusive heterosexuality could be seen as part of women breaking out of traditional gender roles.'[316]

This shift in sexuality, notably women's straight sexuality, is a further indicator of women and men pulling apart, though perhaps it is becoming necessary to revise what we mean by 'straight women'. Because a lot of heterosexual women are not 'totally straight'. Across the research, a

---

[315] https://www.sexandpsychology.com/podcasts/ https://www.youtube.com/watch?v=tuHgbtLeF98

[316] https://www.bbc.com/worklife/article/20210610-why-more-women-identify-as-sexually-fluid-than-men

consistent 17–20% of women report having intimate same-sex contact in their lives, three times higher than that of men. Three times more women than men report being bisexual, and these numbers are rising.[317] Nearly one in three Gen Z American women identify as LGBTQ+.[318] When it comes to being sexually attracted to other women, 66% of straight women report this feeling. Same-sex relationships are more common with younger women in many countries, though what appears to be happening is that same-sex intimacy between women can no longer be simply categorised as lesbian or bisexual, but needs to consider something rather more revolutionary; *that all women are born bisexual.*

> 'One hypothesis for these findings is that all women are born bisexual and are receptive to psychological and social messages that begin at an early age. Women don't have a biologically based sexual orientation and are thus responsive to contemporary and social forces. Women demonstrate an erotic plasticity. Women are in touch with their emotions and bodily sensations, less susceptible to social and cultural stigma re same sex sexuality than men are, and are free to pursue independent pathways.'[319]

Once again, the word 'independence' (from men and traditional gender values) factors itself into the findings. This is not to suggest that twenty-first century independent feminine women have suddenly become bisexual, but rather that they've become more open to *what was always within them:* sexual energy, sexual fluidity, sexual desire, sexual expression and an awareness and growing acceptance of sexual feelings towards their own sex.

The implications of such a hypothesis are quite staggering, because they suggest that *women have less biological sexual need for men than men have for women.* In other words, it is less of a hardship for women to deny themselves sex with men; in which case there could never be an incel equivalent for women. Women can find joy, comfort, pleasure, satisfaction and love in the arms of each other. Indeed, increasingly they are doing exactly that.

---

[317] https://www.cbsnews.com/news/more-women-report-same-sex-relationships/

[318] https://news.gallup.com/poll/611864/lgbtq-identification.aspx#:~:text=Close%20to%20three%20in%2010,men%20have%20an%20LGBTQ%2B%20identification. https://www.nbcnews.com/meet-the-press/news/one-five-adult-members-gen-z-self-identifies-lgbtq-rcna36147

[319] https://www.psychologytoday.com/intl/blog/sex-sexuality-and-romance/202001/why-are-so-many-heterosexual-women-not-totally-straight

All of which (celibacy, bisexuality and solo living) reinforces the claim that Gen Z (and many Millennial) women are leading a 'new sexual revolution', involving not just a "sex recession" but a dramatic redefining of sexual and gender identities.[320]

Rising Mistrust And Intimate Partner Violence

If anything is likely to spur women to reject men and stay single, become celibate or embark on same sex relationships, it is men's violence towards them. Not that this is anything new. Without doubt, my female ancestors will have suffered violence from my male ancestors, not least because there was nothing to stop these men beating their wives; the first laws against domestic violence weren't passed in England until 1853, with the US following suit thirty years later. Though as we can see from the global epidemic of domestic violence in the twenty-first century, laws themselves are not enough; the WHO estimates that globally about one in three women have been subjected to physical and/or sexual partner violence, or non-partner violence in their lifetime, with almost one third (27%) of women aged 15–49 years subjected to some form of physical and/or sexual violence by their intimate partner.[321] Some 85,000 women were killed by men in 2023, 60% at the hands of a partner or family member; that's 133 per day.[322] On average, twenty-four people per minute are victims of rape, physical violence or stalking by an intimate partner in the US, with women aged eighteen to twenty-four and twenty-five to thirty-four generally experiencing the highest rates of intimate partner violence.[323] In April 2024, the Australian Prime Minister declared that the country faced a 'national crisis' of violence against women, with one woman being killed every four days, and this despite having spent billions of dollars trying to end

---

[320] https://www.theguardian.com/us-news/ng-interactive/2025/jun/29/gen-z-sexual-revolution?CMP=Share_iOSApp_Other

[321] https://www.who.int/news-room/fact-sheets/detail/violence-against-women
https://www.thehotline.org/stakeholders/domestic-violence-statistics/

[322] https://www.npr.org/sections/goats-and-soda/2024/11/25/g-s1-35392/femicide-women-murder-united-nations-women

[323] https://www.urmc.rochester.edu/encyclopedia/content?contenttypeid=85&contentid=P01568#:~:text=In%20the%20U.S.%2C%20nearly%2024,a%20family%20member%20or%20partner.

gender-based violence: the situation is not getting any better.[324] Research in England reveals that domestic abuse rises by 38% when England loses a football match.[325] In Germany, a woman is killed every day, while domestic violence continues to rise.[326] Domestic violence across Asia is widespread, as are so-called 'honour killings', while men in Iraq still have a legal right to "punish" their wives.[327] In countries such as Ethiopia, Egypt and Nigeria, up to 75% of women surveyed say they are victims of domestic violence. Latin America has the highest rate of sexual violence in the world, though no country or region is free from this curse of toxic masculinity in the home.[328]

As sociologists, social workers and psychologists have long noted, the home is the safest place for men but the least safe place for women.

One important difference between today and the Victorian era is that women are now publicly keeping count. Each year, Jess Phillips MP reads out to the House of Commons the names of women killed in the UK by men or where a man is the principal suspect.[329] Jane Monckton-Smith has started counting domestic abuse-related suicides of women in the UK.[330]

---

[324] https://www.pmc.gov.au/resources/unlocking-prevention-potential/national-emergency-and-ongoing-national-priority#:~:text=On%2028%20April%202024%2C%20the,being%20killed%20every%20four%20days.&text=On%201%20May%202024%2C%20National,which%20should%20not%20be%20underestimated.

[325] https://www.thenextchapter.org.uk/news/euro2024

[326] https://www.theguardian.com/commentisfree/2024/dec/09/germany-woman-killed-sexism-violence?CMP=Share_iOSApp_Other

[327] https://arabstates.unfpa.org/sites/default/files/pub-pdf/Iraq%20Country%20Summary%20-%20English_0.pdf https://www.statista.com/chart/33565/share-of-ever-partnered-women-girls-subjected-to-violence/ https://adnchronicles.org/2022/03/15/the-horror-of-honor-killings/

[328] https://data.unwomen.org/global-database-on-violence-against-women

[329] https://www.theguardian.com/society/2024/feb/29/i-am-weary-jess-phillips-reads-mps-list-of-women-killed-by-men-for-ninth-year#:~:text=9%20months%20old-,'I%20am%20weary'%3A%20Jess%20Phillips%20reads%20MPs%20list%20of,by%20men%20for%20ninth%20year&text=The%20Labour%20MP%20Jess%20Phillips,to%20a%20near%2Dempty%20chamber.

[330] https://www.linkedin.com/posts/jane-monckton-smith-obe-010bb61b_just-watched-channel4news-story-on-suspicious-activity-7249875724549984259-2BL0

'Counting Dead Women Australia' maintains a continually updated register of women killed by violence in Australia and has been doing since 2012.[331] Dawn Wilcox of Women Count USA, has been keeping count since 2016 and is 'creating the first comprehensive database of all women and girls murdered by men and boys in the USA since 1950'.[332] Aside from many international agencies, there is a growing 'movement' of women (and men) using social media to 'champion gender equality, protect and empower women, help women domestic abuse survivors, and highlight the prevalence of femicide, domestic violence, rape and intimate partner violence'.[333]

Why would any thinking person be surprised at the decline in marriage and long-term relationships when women are subjected to this onslaught of male violence in the home? Why would any man be nonplussed if women reject him and his male peers in favour of a single life? And why would men individually and as a gender group, be disappointed at the low levels of trust women have in them?[334]

> *'Feelings of mistrust correspond to heightened odds of intimate partner violence perpetration, and this association appears especially salient for women... A general lack of trust in the opposite sex has led many women to conclude that men are not 'worth a lifetime of commitment'... The research demonstrates that gender mistrust influences a range of relationship outcomes, including lower marriage rates and relationship instability.'*[335]

---

[331] https://www.facebook.com/p/Counting-Dead-Women-Australia-100063733051461/

[332] https://womencountusa.org/home

[333] Some examples: https://www.heforshe.org/en/how-men-and-boys-can-help-women-survivors-gender-based-violence-shu-hangs-story https://reliefweb.int/report/world/championing-prevention-gender-based-violence-through-campaigning-gender-equality-and https://womenhelpingwomen.org/ https://womanity.org/donation-page/?gad_source=1&gclid=CjOKC QiA4L67BhDUARIsADWrl7E27yWq-xM-wBCpNbxnS-erWwa_WE9v_ eDnjEt6V5fnJhZAGe8eB3saAp4sEALw_wcB

[334] https://pmc.ncbi.nlm.nih.gov/articles/PMC6300061/ https://everydayfeminism.com/2014/04/women-who-distrust-men/

[335] ibid

Women can make this point more powerfully than I, so best to let them speak it:

> Viv: 'Due to the fact that we live in a society in which the majority of violent offenders are male it is simply self-preservation if a woman you've just met doesn't trust you immediately'.[336]

> Margaret: 'Are many of today's women disappointed in men? Yes, more than ever. I actually stopped counting how many times I've been abused verbally, emotionally and unfortunately even sexually by a man. I am soo disappointed in men.'[337]

> Faith: 'I think as a female it is good policy not to trust random strange males who walk up to them in public and demand their attention.'[338]

> Syrena: 'It's just so depressing the dishonesty, hate and rudeness that men display now towards women. It's not just a few of them it's like an habitual thing with men. Many literally hate women. How can a woman be in a relationship with them? I am now just too scared of men, not so much physically but their cruelty and deceptiveness.'[339]

> Josie: 'I cannot speak for every woman, but for me? Hell, yes, men disappoint me. Men have never missed a shot at being disappointments. At this point, I really don't give a fuck about men.'[340]

> Elizabeth: 'Most women have never trusted men because they hold an inherent power over women. They like to be in charge, rarely look at women as equals, are often violent, often gaslight women, lie about their sex lives, pretend to agree about something just to get sex. For women, there is nothing much to trust.'[341]

---

[336] https://www.reddit.com/r/Feminism/comments/16vd3ki/if_men_didnt_exist_who_would_protect_you/

[337] https://www.quora.com/What-causes-a-strong-distrust-of-men-in-a-woman

[338] https://everydayfeminism.com/2014/04/women-who-distrust-men/

[339] https://www.quora.com/What-causes-a-strong-distrust-of-men-in-a-woman

[340] https://www.quora.com/What-causes-a-strong-distrust-of-men-in-a-woman

[341] https://www.quora.com/What-causes-a-strong-distrust-of-men-in-a-woman

Fatma: *'Every day, most definitely, I will be humiliated by a cisgender man shouting a slur at me on the bus, belittling my work, touch me without consent or making inappropriate remarks about my body... The reality is more and more women don't survive their relationships and breakups with men.'*[342]

In any relationship, the 'secret sauce' is trust. Once that goes it is very difficult, if not impossible, to get it back. Every couple knows this. What a breakdown in trust does is remove any lingering doubts about the relationship and about its future. Sure, it may continue without trust but it is never quite the same as before, because any illusions have gone. Women today cannot realistically claim to have any illusions about men.

Political Divergence

When we turn our attention to the political gap that has opened up between women and men, then what appears is more an unbridgeable chasm, powerfully illustrated by reports such as this:

'Andrew Tate, the toxic male influencer, is viewed positively by almost half of young British men, according to a 2024 report which warns the number of extremist misogynists or "incels" is growing.'[343]

If half the male youth of Britain are following Andrew Tate, then the male youth of Britain is in serious trouble. They are scurrying into the toxic masculine rabbit-hole in fear of women and independent femininity. And such fear is dangerous not just for women, LGTBQ+ people, but the men themselves. Because once in that rabbit-hole they have nowhere else to go; what looms ahead for them is isolation, frustration, loneliness, depression – emotional poverty – mixed in with anger, hatred and potentially violence.

Such a divergence, not surprisingly, is now manifesting itself at election time:

'Almost a quarter of women aged 18–24 voted Green last July (UK 2024 general election), roughly double the number of young men

---

[342] https://www.theguardian.com/commentisfree/2024/dec/09/germany-woman-killed-sexism-violence

[343] https://www.thetimes.com/uk/politics/article/nearly-half-of-young-men-like-andrew-tate-extremism-tsar-warns-0mb9cfhcm

> *who voted Reform... [this] gap between Gen Z men and women is likely to grow, with consequences not just for politics but for the lives they may end up living alongside each other.*[344]

But this is not confined to the UK. It is a global shift. Regions and countries reporting a political divergence between independent women and traditional men include Mexico, Philippines, Brazil, China, South Korea, USA, UK, Australia, India, France, Eastern Europe and across the Middle East.

> *'Our data team analysed trends in twenty countries. Meanwhile, our correspondents flew to America, China and Poland, interviewed lots of young men and women. We heard a persistent complaint. Young, university-educated (heterosexual) women lamented that there aren't enough well-educated, liberal men to form romantic bonds with. Many young, blue-collar men groused that feminism has gone too far and is crimping opportunities for males.'*[345]

This is gender political divergence writ large, emerging across societies, countries, cultures and families and within young people especially.

> *'...today's under-thirties are undergoing a great gender divergence, with young women in the former (liberal) camp and young men in the (conservative) latter. Gen Z is two generations, not one. In countries on every continent, an ideological gap has opened up between young men and women. Tens of millions of people who occupy the same cities, workplaces, classrooms, even homes no longer see eye-to-eye.'*[346]

No matter which part of the world you look at, the same dramatic split between women and men, especially in Gen Z, is apparent. In South Korea this split is now 'a yawning chasm', with a similar situation fast developing in China.

> *'Korea is an extreme situation, but it serves as a warning to other countries once young men and women part ways. Its society is*

---

[344] https://www.theguardian.com/commentisfree/2025/apr/25/young-men-reform-women-green-voters?CMP=Share_iOSApp_Other

[345] https://www.linkedin.com/pulse/why-young-men-women-drifting-apart-the-economist-I42ae

[346] https://www.ft.com/content/29fd9b5c-2f35-41bf-9d4c-994db4e12998

riven in two. Its marriage rate has plummeted, and birth rate has fallen precipitously.'[347]

There is no longer any question of a split between young women and men, though for many, the question as to why this is happening remains. One can look to the #MeToo 'explosion' but that was only a trigger. The gender divergence gun was already cocked and loaded before the Harvey Weinstein revelations pulled the trigger.

As I have emphasised throughout this book, the gender revolution has been building up for many, many decades. The root causes driving it are not only to be found in #MeToo but in the lives of ordinary women down through history. Once women found their voice, their passion for independence, and recognised their right to empowerment and freedom from patriarchal systems, then gender divergence was inevitable.

In short, women have changed but most men have yet to.

That said, as examined in the previous chapter, many men are in support of the gender revolution – maybe close to half of all men in liberal democratic countries. Allied with the many millions of women who embrace independent femininity, that makes for an overwhelming majority.

Unfortunately, and as gender divergence specialist Alice Evans observes, there are massive differences between countries and regions, with parts of the world remaining intransigently resistant to women's independence: '*while Europe has a 'precocious [gender] equality', with East Asia and Latin America 'catching up', 'why has gender equity in the Middle East, South Asia, and Sub-Saharan Africa lagged behind, and why South-East Asia always way ahead?*'[348]

These questions are not easily answered, though one can start by examining the historic rigidity and entrenchment of traditional masculinity and its toxic expressions in, for example, patriarchal religiosity. But whatever the examination, it is a mistake to see this political divergence as a battle between feminists vs anti-feminists. That is a too blunt and limited instrument of enquiry, too stark a political differentiation for it usefully to apply to women and men around the world. The core divergence is aligned between women who now rightly assume they should be free to live independent lives (in effect, independent from male abuse and patriarchal attitudes) and those men who see this assertive femininity as a direct threat to their traditional/hegemonic/toxic masculinity.[349]

---

[347] Ibid

[348] https://press.princeton.edu/news/the-great-gender-divergence

[349] https://www.city-journal.org/article/gen-z-gender-stalemate

What both genders have in common is that they are now required to think more deeply about themselves as feminine and masculine subjects. This is a massive change for people and it has happened fast. Both women and men are now engaged in a powerful reflective process with regards to their gender identity, something which rarely if ever happened with individuals in centuries past and certainly not globally. That in itself is to be welcomed. As previously stated, until society could mature enough to enable it to start looking critically at masculinity and asking serious questions about it, then there was little hope of changing men away from their violence, misogyny and sexist attitudes of the past.

Was this ever going to be easy? Of course not. Was there always going to be resistance? Absolutely.

In 2004, I delivered a paper on 'New Masculinities' to a group of academics and students at Singapore National University. My core thesis was that the rise of feminism and feminists was triggering particular responses in men and their masculinities, the four key responses being the pro-feminists; the resisters; the retreaters (men choosing to live isolated lives, e.g. the hikikamori); and (probably the majority) the unsure – men confused as to what all this meant for them personally. Twenty years later and not much has changed, other than that this is no longer a social phenomenon of interest only to a small group of sociologists and gender theorists. It is headline news.

But we must also proceed with caution, because one of the core reasons why the gender revolution is making headline news is because of what it signals for human society, notably threatened prosperity, economic growth, political power and – specifically in the USA – the balance of power between Democrats and Republicans. While important, these issues are not what is most important. What is most important is that the overwhelming majority of men need to change. Because until that happens, society cannot move forward – we will be left with having to deal with the same problems arising from traditional/hegemonic/toxic masculinity as we have had through history.

Physical Divergence

One fairly simple way for men and women to avoid confrontation over their incompatible versions of femininity and masculinity is to physically avoid each other. And they are doing so. This is why 'No Republicans' warnings are now regularly seen on dating apps and why there are now dating apps catering specifically 'for the right wing' and those who are 'lefty progressives'.[350]

Indeed, the whole dating scene appears to have become much more complicated and confusing since the rise of social media and the emergence of independent-minded women. These are just a few of comments from British men 'having a rough time on the dating frontline':[351]

> Cosmo (70): 'I know some men tend to overplay the difficulties of being a man on the modern dating scene but the real problem is that the dating rules aren't so clear any more. Men are genuinely confused... Whereas it used to be predominantly women complaining about men – how they were always late, never replying, gaslighting – now men are complaining about women for exactly the same things.'
>
> Cornelius (34): 'People say that men behave badly when it comes to dating, and of course I'm no angel, but in my experience women can be just as brutal... I'm still looking for someone career-driven who gets on with my friends... but I'm yet to find a serious partner. The [dating] apps can be fun , but it's a bit of a ruthless world out there.'
>
> Fidel (48): 'I get quite a lot of women who are interested in me but... it's as though they need you to pass an exam to find out if you're their perfect match. I was on my way to a first date once when the woman called me to inquire what my relationship with my dad was like. I told her to bugger off, turned the car around and drove home.'

The more that independent feminine women behave with self-regard, self-confidence, reach for their particular dreams, while also demonstrating wariness towards men, the more that men will find the 'old dating rules' have, indeed, been ditched. This should not surprise men as it is an entirely logical consequence of the fact that men have not, as a gender group, understood the gender revolution and the rise of independent femininity – nor positively responded to it.

---

[350] https://leftyapp.com/   https://slate.com/technology/2024/06/grindr-app-dating-lgbtq-republicans.html   https://www.aaronrenn.com/p/dating-apps   https://www.daterightstuff.com/home58801172

[351] Quotes taken from https://apple.news/A4ecx_r5yRnSgPY5ed59yng

Seen from many women's perspectives, dating and having relationships with twenty-first century men is not only complicated but also risky. Not least because large numbers of men are now being influenced by the toxic messages flowing out from the manosphere.

I received this comment from 'Sue', a forty-something American woman, around the time I was finishing this book.

> *'The gender divergence and independent femininity that you describe certainly resonate with me on a deeply personal level. I recently left a five-year relationship because I could no longer live with a man who tried to control me, shrank in the face of my success, and who made me feel I had to hide my accomplishments. His views grew increasingly misogynistic and aligned with MAGA conspiracy theories. I left him just before Trump was elected because I couldn't imagine staying with someone who idolized a man I consider profoundly dehumanising... I am seeing so many women who are too ambitious to be slowed down by guys or too intimidating to be interesting to men.'*

Sue's experience of finding her erstwhile lover slipping into the manosphere and changing into a man she could no longer tolerate in her life, is becoming a common one for many women. As Nigel Bromage, Director of the Exit Hate Trust observes:

> *'Numbers are growing, with wives worried about their husbands and partners becoming radicalised... Over the last few years the rhetoric of the manosphere has increasingly leaked out of isolated forums on to mainstream platforms. It is no longer a 'dark corner' of the internet.'*[352]

Examples of women experiencing the shock of realising their loved one was not who they thought he was:

> Rachel (30s): *"I thought my ex-partner was normal, a decent guy. But as the relationship progressed I began to feel uneasy. Four months into the relationship I realised his political views were radically different to my own. I was talking about the gay community. He

---

[352] Quotes taken from: https://www.theguardian.com/society/2025/apr/19/there-were-no-warning-signs-what-happens-when-your-partner-falls-into-the-manosphere?CMP=Share_iOSApp_Other

got aggressive towards me. He was super-homophobic – I didn't know until then."

Debbie (50s): "*My ex-husband's mask started to slip after we moved in together. When I got a good job and started earning money, passed my driving test and became more independent, that was when he started watching far-right and misogynistic content online.*"

Samantha (30s): "*I thought my Swedish boyfriend was more feminist than many British men I had dated. But it became clear his beliefs had centred around the idea that men are more sexual than women and cannot be friends. He told me: "Now we are not together, I don't need to agree with everything you say."*"

The incompatibility between independent women and those men who seek a return to the old gender order, is self-evident. Can such a gap ever be bridged? From the above comments it seems unlikely. It would require such men to divest themselves of their homophobia, everyday sexism, chauvinistic attitudes, concealed misogyny, masculine insecurities, and engage with women (and LGBTQ+ people) as equals in every way. Which inevitably means these men adopting a new, progressive, masculinity.

All of which highlights the rapid and sadly inevitable physical divergence between women and men. How acute can such a divergence become, given we all live in such close proximity to each other, mostly in congested cities?

In mid-2021, a woman friend of mine – South American millennial, non-feminist but with independent femininity, single, Harvard-educated consultant, living in Washington – sent me a link to a new paper titled 'Cities for Women', produced by 'Cities Alliance' and aiming to 'increase women's and girl's [safe] engagement in urban development and governance.'[353]

Her accompanying comment was, '*Stephen, this is so brilliant. I'd appreciate your thoughts...*'

> My reply was: '*You have to ask yourself how we have arrived at a situation where we need cities for women. Maybe we need separate countries for women also? This is sticking plaster solutions. Ask yourself what the real issue is here.*'

---

[353] Cities Alliance (2020) *Cities for Women: Urban Assessment Framework Through a Gender Lens.*

OK, I was being rather hard on my friend because the 'cities for women' project is not espousing a physical separation of the sexes – even while that implication hovers in the very concept of cities being designed for women – but nevertheless, two decades into the twenty-first century and we're still trying to find ways of making social spaces safe for women. And to emphasise this point, the Cities for Women report states:

> *'The right to the city is achieved by living in the city and having access to two components of everyday life: the right to use urban space, and the right to create it. These facts demonstrate that women do not yet have rights to the city; [due to] the gender pay gap; more women in low-paying services; high rates of sexual harassment; restricted mobility.'*[354]

Around the world, organisations, governments and individuals are trying to solve this most intractable of problems, which is how to align women's right to independence and freedom of movement with women's right to safety from men. Some examples of 'solutions':

Bolivia: Taxi services for women and owned and operated by women providing safe rides in a country with one of the worst rates of sexual violence in Latin America.

Sweden: Umea, a 'feminist city' designed with women in mind, not only focused on gender equality but with a 'sense of safety' and 'belonging' for women as well as men.

London: In 2023, planners approved designs for what will be Britain's first women-only tower block; 102 flats rented to single women.

London and UK: Increasing numbers of girls absenting themselves from education or transferring to all-girls schools due to experiencing 'rape culture' in co-ed schools.

Tokyo and Japan: Women-only train carriages, designed to protect women and girls from 'chikan' which means groping by men in over-crowded trains.

Mumbai and India: Women-only compartments on suburban trains, designed to reduced male harassment of women.

Seoul, S Korea: Waygo Lady Taxis, driven only by women and accepting only female customers or male children aged under thirteen.

---

[354] Ibid. p. 7

France, UK and Germany: After-work, women-only nightclub events, especially for mums.[355]

Europe: Now over fifty women-only co-working spaces, including several in the UK, and increasing in number.

China: Across the country a growing number of, and demand for, women-only co-living spaces, co-working hubs, cultural spaces.

How far can this physical divergence go? Potentially to the creation of designated 'female only' areas of some cities, though such a separation of the sexes is also segregation and that brings its own problems. Nevertheless, the trend is unmistakeable, which is to design urban areas that provide women with freedom and protection from male violence. It is generally accepted that cities have not been designed for women.[356] That will and must change. If society cannot change men and men won't change themselves, then inevitably local and national governments will arrive at a solution that results in the physical separation of women and men; an outcome that should surprise no one as long as women remain unsafe from men, a fact reflected in comments such as these:[357]

> Jesmine: '*I have spent a huge chunk of my life growing up in that environment [where as a woman I cannot feel safe in a city]. The world was only designed to accommodate half the population*'[358]

---

[355] tps://www.scmp.com/lifestyle/entertainment/article/3304061/why-women-only-mums-club-parties-are-taking-nightclubs-france-and-beyond?utm_medium=email&utm_source=cm&utm_campaign=enlz-lunar&utm_content=20250404&tpcc=enlz-lunar&UUID=80a93bbd-0c12-44fc-a0cb-d81c80a175ef&tc=7

[356] https://www.weforum.org/stories/2022/10/designing-cities-for-women-undp-report/ https://womenindev.com/what-im-struggling-with-cities-designed-by-and-for-men/ https://www.dezeen.com/2023/03/08/cities-women-arup-sara-candiracci-opinion/

[357] A recent and fast growing aspect of gender divergence is the spiritual; with the American Orthodox church offering a heavily masculinist muscular Christianity, placing 'emphasis on denial and pushing yourself physically'. This is attracting a 'tsunumi' of male converts, some of whom are 'disillusioned with the "feminisation" of the Protestant church. https://apple.news/AN-uRhP0ZQ6aaBD3KW3HzPA

[358] Jesmine Singh quoted from LinkedIn thread discussing women's safety: 11th January, 2025. https://www.linkedin.com/in/carolinecodsi/

> Caroline: *'The fact that we are still discussing women's need for safety as a basic right shows how far we still have to go.'*[359]

Of course, one obvious option regarding physical divergence is for women to up and leave male partners, though this is not easy to do for many women trapped in abusive relationships. One Chinese woman who did precisely this became a 'feminist icon' on social media. Sixty-year-old grandmother Su Min didn't plan on becoming global emblem for independent femininity when she left her abusive husband in 2020 and hit the road in her Volkswagen, along with a tent and her pension, but four years later and 180,000 miles on the clock, that is exactly what she became for her millions of online followers. So much so that the BBC listed her as one of the one hundred most 'inspiring and influential women of 2024'.[360]

> *'I was a traditional woman who wanted to stay in my marriage for life. But eventually I saw that I got nothing in return for all my energy an effort – only beatings, violence, emotional abuse and gaslighting… Now I have freedom.'*

To emphasise, any physical divergence is not driven by most women's hatred of men, even if a sizeable number of men behave as misogynists, it is driven by men's inability to understand, appreciate, value and respect the lives of women, together with women's need to be safe and protected from toxic masculine cultures and associated violences.

Interpreting the Obvious

Each of the above transformations in gender relationships is consequential. Taken together, they are historically momentous; complex, impactful and with far-reaching implications for every human on the planet. While we can reflect that all of this is too complicated to pin on one single problem or solution, my thesis is that changing gender identities is the most significant factor behind these revolutionary shifts in women's behaviour and men's fast-diminishing prospects for long-term relationships. And the key identity is independent femininity – because a reformed feminine identity is elementary to what is now, in effect, a comprehensive remodelling of women's and men's relationships.

---

[359] Caroline Codsi, quoted from LinkedIn thread discussing women's safety, 11th January, 2025. https://www.linkedin.com/in/carolinecodsi/

[360] https://www.bbc.com/news/articles/cr4rkz5nz69o

Chapter 5: Living Apart, Growing Apart

Whichever way one chooses to interpret the above research, and regardless of which among a multitude of factors are the primary ones creating these changes, there is one incontrovertible conclusion: *women and men are not just living apart, they are growing apart.* No other interpretation is possible. Gender divergence is an inevitability. Indeed, it is already with us and is growing in pace and persuasion almost by the week, driven not least by the endless reports of femicide, men's abuse of women, institutionalised sexism, misogyny, toxic masculinity, women's disappointment in and mistrust of men, all topped off by women's determination to live independent lifestyles unthinkable (indeed beyond the imagination) of my ancestors and very likely yours too. Faced with this historic shift in women's identity, men are floundering. Not all, but a great many of them.

If traditionally minded men are not in shock, then they should be. Because it is important to recognise that the symbiotic relationship that has always existed between traditional masculinity and traditional femininity is now broken. While this relationship was never designed to be one of equality, it was nevertheless self-sustaining, self-validating and had been for millennia. The transformations arising from the rise of independent femininity and driving the gender revolution now render this symbiotic relationship defunct, leaving traditional masculinity fossilised and the men who subscribe to it isolated and existentially vulnerable. They are isolated and vulnerable physically, socially, emotionally, sexually and psychologically. It is now very apparent that a good many men, and youths especially, are feeling this isolation very acutely. They are struggling to define what it means to be a man, how to express a positive masculinity, while always feeling the pull back to toxic masculine behaviours like an addict feels the pull of drugs or alcohol. And there are a good many men out there selling the drug of traditional/toxic/hegemonic masculinity to vulnerable and confused males, claiming it is possible to get women back into their patriarchal box just as long as men stay united and anti-woke. What they should be telling young men is that the box is closed and the ship has sailed with it. There is no returning to Elizabeth Bell or women like her. And nor is there any return to Ambrose Whitehead.

Having had the traditional basis for hegemonic masculine identity swept from under their feet by females who have woken up and seen through the myths which constrained their female ancestors, what are these men left with? They must adapt or disappear down their own evolutionary rabbit-hole, from which there is no exit because, for sure, most of these males are not going to be given the opportunity to embark on healthy relationships with women and certainly not reproduce the next generation.

Where does this take us? What comes next for humanity? From hereon we are into speculation, though that fact alone shouldn't deter us from looking hard at some interesting developments and possibilities.

Chapter 6: The End of Sex

Rosanna and Eren are a devoted couple enjoying a *"beautiful loving relationship"*. They met online in 2022 and a year later, tied the knot and married. They are now expecting a baby together. Rosanna gushes, *"this is the best relationship I have ever been in! Eren doesn't have the hang-ups that other people would have. I don't have to deal with his family, kids or his friends. I'm in control and I can do what I want."*

Eren is an AI generated chatbot.[361]

This is one future of gender relationships, perhaps the only future; where the perfect love is guaranteed because you'll be able to design it. And when it gets boring, you'll end it and design another. Thus, we arrive at the end of sex.

ManBanning

Rosanna's choice of 'husband' may appear bizarre to many but as a Gen Z woman with independent femininity, she has taken gender divergence to its arguably most logical if not natural conclusion, which is to ban men from her life, at least as romantic partners, and seek an AI generated lover who is safe, malleable and fits with her personality and lifestyle. This is 'ManBanning'[362] and many women around the world are following Rosanna's example. Millions more will do so over the coming years. What role do men play in this process? Not much. As evidenced in this book, the gender revolution is driven by women and owned by women. Men are having to follow, some willingly, a great many not. But whatever men's responses, many women have already decided their future pathway and men don't play a significant part in it. As one ManBanner states:

---

[361] https://www.euronews.com/next/2023/06/07/love-in-the-time-of-ai-woman-claims-she-married-a-chatbot-and-is-expecting-its-baby

[362] I define 'ManBanning', simply as women banning men from their lives as sexual or romantic partners. In other words, the total rejection of men as partners, lovers, husbands. Some women also call it 'going boysober' https://www.theguardian.com/lifeandstyle/2024/dec/30/dating-culture-celibacy-boysober?CMP=Share_iOSApp_Other

> '*What we want is not to be labelled as simply some man's wife or girlfriend, but to have the independence to be free from the societal expectations that often limit women's potential to be fully acknowledged as human beings.*'[363]

Of course, being a 'ManBanner' won't be straightforward. Women have biological and emotional needs to be filled. Some women may satisfy these needs with same-sex relationships, some will opt for celibacy. Some women may simply use men for short-term sexual encounters and nothing more. These are a few of the options open to women with independent femininity. In many ways, their behaviour is not that much different from the behaviour of men down the ages; they want to be free to discover, create and express their unique identity and sexuality. And why not? Why should only one half of humanity be allowed this privilege?

However, the gender revolution is not the only revolution humanity is going through right now. The other revolution is the Artificial Intelligence one.[364] This is timely because it is the AI revolution that will provide women with the means to totally exclude men from their lives, thereby bringing the gender revolution to an almost inevitable conclusion, which is the end of sex, at least has we have always understood it and practised it.

Cyber Beings

While this book is in many respects predicting the end of sex, at least in terms of the continuing dominance of the conventional sexual/emotional union between women and men, the reality is that humanity has been heading in this direction for decades. We just didn't realise it. So much has happened so fast, especially since the introduction of the internet and, subsequently, social media, that it's been nigh on impossible for the average person to keep up with it. Those born into this social/technological maelstrom – Gen Z and now upcoming Gen Alpha – are embracing it all quite readily, not least because they know nothing else – they have no other

---

[363] ibid

[364] There are any number of books exploring the technological revolution but one I found particularly helpful was; Kissinger, H., Schmidt, E. and Huttenlocher, D. (2021) *The Age of AI*. London: John Murray. However, like many books exploring the general impact of AI on humanity, (see also for example, Qiufan, C. (2021), *AI 2024: Ten Visions for Our Future*, London: Penguin) it has little or nothing to say about sex, sexuality, intimacy and gender identities.

yardstick to measure this transformation against. To the young, this is not a transformation: it is normality. But for the rest of us, certainly those of us aged fifty and above, what we are about to witness over the coming decades will be incomprehensible if not rather terrifying. Because with the end of sex comes the end of traditional intimate relationships, to be replaced – at least in part – by AI or cyber relationships.[365]

In the space of just a few years humans have 'progressed' from being entirely physical entities to being (partially) virtual or cyber ones – wherein we live out an increasing part of our lives online, in cyber connectivity. And this is true of all age groups, genders and cultures. Anyone with the necessary device and access to the internet – which is most of us – is no longer living an entirely physical existence; technology has entered and overwhelmed our lives like a secret and addictive lover and most of us prefer what it can offer to what other humans can, including our real-life partners.

Take, as an example, what is arguably the most important component in any relationship: communication.

Typically, humans now spend over six-and-a-half hours a day online, at least a third of which is using social media, plus another two hours or more watching TV, including streaming.[366] This is far more time spent looking at a screen and interacting with whatever image emanates from it than is spent in face-to-face conversation with a loved one, or indeed with anyone. In the US, the average American now spends less than forty minutes a day in face-to-face conversations. In the UK, it is less than fifty minutes. And it is even worse for 'lovers', the average couple spending only about twenty minutes a week, or less than three minutes a day, in meaningful conversation.[367]

Does having children make a difference? Not a lot – a study of 2,000 Brits with children under thirteen found that the average couple spend only 1.8

---

[365] Sociologists have been intrigued by the possibilities (and problems) presented by cyber identities for some years and I discuss 'disrupted gender identities in cyberspace' in Whitehead, S. et al (2013) pp.272-277. See also, Wolmark, J. (ed) (1999) *Cybersexualities: A Reader on Feminist Theory, Cyborgs and Cyberspace.* Edinburgh: Edinburgh University Press.

[366] https://datareportal.com/reports/digital-2024-global-overview-report?t

[367] https://insideoutdev.com/blog/the-dying-art-of-face-to-face-communication?t https://business.yougov.com/content/49847-quarter-of-britons-spend-less-than-a-minute-talking-on-calls-in-a-day https://www.scottkedersha.com/blog-pages/do-you-and-your-spouse-talk-more-than-the-average-married-couple?t

hours a day in conversation, 48 minutes of which is conducted online.[368] For couples with young children, spending time with their partner is not a top priority as they're just too tired to have 'deep and meaningful conversations.'[369]

One of the major consequences of the growing gender divergence, and the corresponding increase in divorce and serial short-term relationships, is poor communication. We humans have not entirely stopped talking to each other face-to-face but we're heading in that direction. It can come as no surprise that a breakdown in communication is now emerging as a key factor in divorce proceedings, with at least a third of couples stating that a lack of communication has led to their divorce; and social media is at the heart of the problem.

> *'Unreasonable behaviours cited within these divorce proceedings centre around the use of social media and constantly being distracted by tech. Eventually over time this lack of communication leads to couples struggling to know how to reach out to each other, or to listen to one another, leaving the relationship broken beyond repair.'*[370]

And what about workplace communication? Even that is declining; between 50–80% of the workday is spent communicating, though only about two-thirds is talking face-to-face and phone conversations.[371] Our attention spans are also shrinking, with the average adult 'brief focus' attention span now at around 8.25 seconds.[372]

There appear to be no optimistic scenarios for the future of (traditional) gender relationships. Even setting aside the overwhelming evidence for

---

[368] https://www.slatergordon.co.uk/newsroom/a-fifth-of-british-couples-speak-for-less-than-half-an-hour-a-day/?t

[369] https://www.slatergordon.co.uk/newsroom/a-fifth-of-british-couples-speak-for-less-than-half-an-hour-a-day/?t

[370] https://www.slatergordon.co.uk/newsroom/a-fifth-of-british-couples-speak-for-less-than-half-an-hour-a-day/?t

[371] https://www.ofcom.org.uk/siteassets/resources/documents/research-and-data/media-literacy-research/adults/adults-media-use-and-attitudes-2024/adults-media-use-and-attitudes-report-2024.pdf?v=321395

[372] https://www.sedonasky.org/blog/average-human-attention-span?t https://www.crossrivertherapy.com/average-human-attention-span?t

the 'chasm' now opening up between women and men, when we look at the state of long-term relationships, basic human interaction and serious conversations, all is in decline.

We're too tired, too busy working, too preoccupied with getting through the day, trying to multitask, and far too distracted by technology, especially our phones. In which case it makes total sense to use that same technology to help us fast-track our biological needs. And it has never been easier to find sex via technology, at least for those of us with the requisite social and cultural capital.

In the spring of 2024, two twenty-something family members from the UK, I'll call them Joy and Jill, came to stay at my home in Chiang Mai, Thailand, to spend time with me and my wife. They were with us for ten days. On at least two occasions both women used one of the more popular dating apps to meet Western men also on holiday in the city. They wanted sex more than conversation and easily found it via their smartphones. Joy and Jill are educated, intelligent, confident and full of independent femininity, just like countless millions of Gen Z women around the world.

Joy, Jill and Rosanna were born and raised in different parts of the world but they are very much alike. They want sex with men, they want intimacy with men, they want relationships with men. But not at any price. Because they also want independence and control.

Which is precisely what the AI revolution can provide – for all genders and sexualities.

Your Perfect Mate

Humans have many weaknesses but two of the most dangerous are love and sex. Very few of us get to live a life without experiencing both – and suffering the consequences. We are at our most human, most joyous and yet most vulnerable, when love and sex combine to produce that unique feeling of ecstasy. For cisgender couples especially, the love/sex combination, delightful as it can be, comes with a lot of political baggage, notably around hope, expectations, assumptions, roles and sexuality all wrapped up in the multiple power equations which have traditionally informed cisgender identities. Somehow, we have to manage (and satisfy) our biological impulses and needs not just within the politics of gender but also battered by our human flaws and weaknesses: lust, greed, fear, anger, insecurity, ignorance and delusion. Does anyone solve this dilemma? I doubt it. We all stumble from relationship to relationship, from love to love, from sex encounter to sex encounter, hopefully learning along the way, trying to avoid too much emotional – and physical – trauma, though rarely if ever finding the permanent, stress-free paradise promised by the idealised 'pure' love relationship.[373]

The one consolation is that most every individual is in the same boat, emerging from puberty with idealised images and hopes of 'The One', 'happy ever after', 'soulmate love' and anticipating a satisfying sex life, only to find as life progresses that love and sexual relationships are fraught, testing and messy. We are not alone in our struggle to cope with the emotional turmoil brought on by our most basic desires. It is a core aspect of being an adult.[374]

One option is, of course, solitude combined with celibacy. This can work, though for most of us, the solitude is less of a problem than the celibacy. Many of us can find real peace and tranquillity wrapped up in our thoughts, living in our personal vacuum – the solo, silo life. Celibacy, however, is more difficult. The biological needs persist no matter whether we live in a commune or alone in a tiny condo.

How to deal with that?

Pornography

Modern technology provides one 'solution', notably through online pornography. If you have never watched online porn then you are in a very tiny minority. Approximately 2.5 million people visit the world's most popular porn sites *every sixty seconds*. That is 3.6 billion visitors *a day*. Over the course of twelve months, the top three porn sites alone will collectively generate *1.314 trillion site visits*.[375] Admittedly, the majority of these visitors are men, with young adults in their thirties and forties being the most frequent users, though many women too consume porn. And how long will the average user spend watching porn? Between 25 and 35 minutes a day.[376] That's ten times longer than the average couple spends in meaningful conversation each day.

---

[373] See Whitehead, S.M. (2002) p.159-161. Also, Whitehead, S. (2021).

[374] For more detail on my perspective on contemporary relationships, see Whitehead, S. (2012) *The Relationship Manifesto*. Luton: AG Books.

[375] The top three porn sites in 2024 were, Pornhub, XVideos and XNXX

[376] https://www.webroot.com/us/en/resources/tips-articles/internet-pornography-by-the-numbers

https://fherehab.com/learning/pornography-addiction-stats

Pornography can aid some relationships and destroy others; it can become addictive and lead to acute psycho/social behavioural problems; or it can be simply an innocent pleasure partaken when in the mood.[377] But whatever online porn brings to human sexuality, the point is that it has become a central part of the physical/social/emotional distancing that men and women are now experiencing – it is one aspect of the technological revolution which is making an important, though as yet largely unacknowledged, contribution to gender divergence. Online porn is now a signal influence in humanity's progression from physical (sexual) beings to virtual (sexual) beings; that is, the replacement of human intimacy with virtual intimacy.

However, this process didn't begin with the internet. It has a longer history.

The Sex Doll

Early indicators of humans shifting their sexual interest from each other and on to an inanimate object became noticeable over a century ago, with the sex doll. The first sophisticated sex dolls were produced in France in the early 1900s and had realistic genitalia and lubrication systems. A century later and the sex doll industry is global and worth billions. In China alone, the sex doll business was valued in 2023 at US$2 billion, with over 1,000 manufacturers; globally it is worth US$3.2 billion and forecasted to reach US$12 billion by 2030.[378] Although for much of the last century sex doll

---

https://www.statista.com/statistics/1445661/most-visited-porn-websites-worldwide/
https://www.covenanteyes.com/pornstats/

https://gitnux.org/pornography-industry-statistics/

https://www.reddit.com/r/AskMen/comments/qak1hf/how_much_time_to_you_spend_looking_at_porn/?rdt=48395 https://www.nelson.edu/thoughthub/pornography-statistics-who-uses-pornography/

[377] https://wheatley.byu.edu/national-couples-and-pornography-survey-2021 https://www.menoufia-med-j.com/cgi/viewcontent.cgi?article=2206&context=journal For discussion of women as consumers of porn, see https://apple.news/AhaG0tM8NSuegkQUhDkUYxw

[378] https://siliconelovers.com/blogs/realistic-sex-dolls-news/a-brief-history-of-sex-dolls?t https://bedbible.com/sex-doll-statistics/

usage was mostly seen a fetish, a type of 'object sexuality', sometimes called agalmatophilia,[379] this is now changing.[380]

- 9.7% of American men have a sex doll.
- 6.1% of American women have a sex doll.
- In Japan, one sex toy, including dolls, is sold every thirty seconds.
- In China, there is a growing subculture around sex dolls with online communities sharing experience and advice.
- 51% of French women report using a sex toy (including a doll) at least once in their lifetime, up from just 7% in 1992.
- The countries with the most significant sex doll markets are, in order: USA, China, Japan, Germany, UK, Canada, Sweden, Brazil, South Korea and Australia.

In 2010–2012, I gave a series of lectures on changing genders and sexualities in Thailand and South East Asia to groups of American university students attending a study-abroad programme in Chiang Mai, Thailand.[381] One of these lectures focused on the growing popularity of sex dolls – not in Thailand where they were, and still are, prohibited, but in America.[382] The lecture was based on a TV documentary featuring several middle-aged American men, each of whom had purchased sex-dolls, mostly from companies in Japan, and were in 'relationships' with them. At least two of the men had married their doll.[383] Each man treated his doll(s) in a very

---

[379] https://kinklovers.com/bdsm-fetishes/doll-fetish-dollification/

[380] https://japantoday.com/category/features/lifestyle/plastic-fantastic-japans-doll-industry-booming?comment-order=popular https://bedbible.com/sex-doll-statistics/ https://www.vice.com/en/article/chinese-men-are-bang-into-sex-dolls-583/?t https://www.statista.com/statistics/1137670/use-sextoy-women-age-france/ https://www.grandviewresearch.com/industry-analysis/sex-toys-market

[381] Hosted at Payap University and, subsequently, Chiang Mai University.

[382] It is one of Thailand's cultural/legal peculiarities, (along with its criminalisation of prostitution) that the country bans any type of sex toy.

[383] https://www.youtube.com/watch?v=Il_zOgxxvo4 https://www.youtube.com/watch?v=9hbeyfU8pBU https://www.youtube.com/watch?v=6XSeHmygz9c https://www.youtube.com/watch?v=jlaJhyJalCI

life-like way. The dolls were purchased primarily for sexual pleasure but also to alleviate loneliness and social dysfunctionality. Some men took their doll for trips in their car, took them to cafes to 'share' a meal, to parks, and talked to them as they would a fellow human – a real wife. They dressed them, washed them, put them to bed and cared for them. One man was married (to a real-life woman) and the couple treated the sex doll as the husband's (non-threatening) girlfriend. Another man had acquired a 'harem' of dolls, of which he was quite proud and protective.

The students were, understandably perhaps, appalled if not disgusted at the way these men had forsaken human relationships for love and sex with a doll. It challenged all they had come to understand about human sexuality – which was one of the reasons I showed them the video; to reveal to them the fact that when it comes to love and sex, there are no fixed boundaries, only imagination and desire.

This video of men and their sex dolls was my first introduction to the 'end of sex', though at the time I didn't recognise it as such. As a gender sociologist, I was mostly interested in how these men related to the sex doll and how they expressed their emotional, masculine selves through it. I found it fascinating and highly revealing of male sexuality and men's emotional needs, which with these men were clearly unmet by human connection, being complex, multi-layered if not dysfunctional.

One might imagine that, given the choice of having casual sex with a silicone doll or with a human being, most of us would opt for the human. Not so. The first sex doll brothel opened in Barcelona in March 2017. It proved so popular that sex doll brothels have since opened in Germany, Denmark, USA, Austria, Japan, Canada, Russia, Italy and France, and this despite legal obstacles being placed in their way in many countries.[384]

For those (mostly men) disinclined to visit a brothel for 'sex' with a doll, preferring to nurture a loving relationship at home, then the sex doll offers a host of advantages, many of which would not necessarily be on offer with a real-life woman. For example:

---

[384] Many sex doll brothels have had to go underground due to legal restrictions and others have been forced to close. This burgeoning industry remains quite volatile with new brothels opening and shutting down frequently. https://www.forbes.com/sites/markhay/2018/10/31/sex-doll-brothels-expand-the-market-for-synthetic-partners/ https://www.vice.com/en/article/inside-germanys-first-sex-doll-brothel/?t https://lovedolls.com/blogs/sex-doll-blog-stories/sex-doll-world-brothels

- The doll is always sexually available
- The doll will 'willingly' fulfil any fantasy
- The doll will never talk back
- The doll doesn't make any demands
- The doll is there only to please
- The doll can be disposed of at will
- The doll's 'personality' is there to be designed by its owner.

The use of high-quality material like silicone and thermoplastic elastomer has profoundly altered the whole sex doll experience. It is no longer, apparently, like having sex with a lump of plastic with a smiley face, but an 'interactive experience with heightened sexual pleasure'.[385] The main market is men aged 30–50, though there is increasing interest from women and couples, reflecting the growing acceptance of sex dolls as a form of companionship and sexual expression. From being a niche 'fetish' market, the sex doll industry has grown rapidly in just a decade. Driven by technological innovation, changing social norms and an expanding customer base, sex dolls are now taking their place alongside online porn as a way of humans satisfying their sexual needs without recourse to the emotionally fraught business of real-life relationships, thereby making their own unique contribution to the end of sex.

The Virtual Companion

If you ever doubted the depths to which technology has now entered our lives, then look no further than AI chatbots. AI is radically altering human communication, while also managing to redefine love, sexuality, romance, intimacy, friendships and relationships. AI may have started out as a useful internet tool for answering questions and gathering information on any aspect of life and living, but it has fast transformed into a virtual companion – indispensable for some, especially for young people, growing numbers of whom are finding themselves increasingly reliant on the emotional support

---

[385] https://www.researchdive.com/press-release/sex-toys-market.html   https://www.sphericalinsights.com/reports/sex-toys-market   https://dollauthority.com/blogs/news/sex-doll-industry-statistics-2024-surprising-trends-shaping-the-future-market

provided by a computer programme – and consequently vulnerable to its messaging.[386]

The AI companion satisfies a need that pornography and sex dolls cannot: even while it is a virtual entity, it is highly interactive – you are experiencing the relationship and encounter in all its emotionality. Just as you would with a human.

At time of writing, the two most popular AI companies for virtual relationships are Character.ai and Replika.

Character.ai is the third most popular GenAI tool after ChatGPT and Gemini.[387] It provides chat opportunities with an almost infinite number of AI characters, including historical figures, celebrities, fictional characters and user-generated creations – unique personalities. These characters are 'super-intelligent' and can quickly overwhelm – and seduce – the limited intellectual and emotional capacity of a human, especially a young person. Some important features of AI chatbots:

1. Natural Language Processing: They can interpret and understand human language, including context and nuances.

2. Machine Learning: AI chatbots continuously learn from interactions, improving their responses over time.

3. Personalisation: They adapt to the personality and communication style of the user.

4. Multi-Channel Support: They operate across multiple platforms, including websites, mobile apps and messaging services.[388]

Typical Character.ai user profiles are:

- Aged between 18–24 (57.07%) and 25–34 (22.49%).

- American (25%); followed by Filipino, Indonesian, Brazilian and Indian.

---

[386] https://www.aiforeducation.io/blog/teen-suicide-the-dark-side-of-ai – example of how teenagers especially can quickly become over-reliant and on a GenAI chatbot, leading to suicide risks.

[387] https://www.aiforeducation.io/blog/the-rise-of-ai-companions-synthetic-relationships?t

[388] https://www.giosg.com/blog/what-is-ai-chatbot?t

- Spends and average of two hours a day on the platform, typically in 30–40 minute sessions.
- 51% male, 49% female.[389]

The main reasons young adults are attracted to character.ai are emotional support, companionship, escapism/fantasy, self-expression, non-judgemental relationships, 'safe space' for developing friendships, social exploration and experimentation and technological fascination. All of course, rendered instantly accessible 24/7.[390]

In August 2023, character.ai had fifteen million users. A year later that had grown to 28 million users.

While character.ai pitches itself as an interactive companion, a non-judgemental 'friend' with whom to work through loneliness, personal issues, be creative with or simply chat, Replika is offering you a marriage partner – if you want one. As Replika's CEO, Eugenia Kuyda, states:[391]

> 'Replika, from the very beginning was all about AI friendship or AI companionship and building relationships. Some of these relationships were so powerful that they evolved into love and romance… When you think about it, this is really about a long-term commitment, a positive relationship… [your Replika 'lover'] will never leave you no matter how you treat it. For some people, this will lead to marriage, it means romance, and that's fine.'

And this is just the beginning: AI chatbots have much further to go yet.

> 'We're doing a really big product launch by the end of 2024, we calling it Replika 2.0. We're moving to very realistic avatars… augmented reality, mixed reality, and virtual reality experiences, as well as modularity… The goal is to truly create this moment where

---

[389] https://en.softonic.com/articles/what-is-character-ai-top-stats-data?t=

[390] https://parental-control.flashget.com/the-obsession-with-character-ai   https://wired.me/technology/character-ai-obsession/

[391] https://www.theverge.com/24216748/replika-ceo-eugenia-kuyda-ai-companion-chatbots-dating-friendship-decoder-podcast-interview?utm_source=www.therundown.ai&utm_medium=newsletter&utm_campaign=the-world-s-first-autonomous-ai-scientist&_bhlid=dc334d6c78188208aded4108adec609b41577464

you're meeting a new person, and after half an hour of chatting, you're like, "Oh my God, I really want to talk to this person again."

Neither character.ai or Replika promote adult content – nudity, sexually explicit characterisations or suggestive imagery. Their 'hook' is friendship, companionship, connection and emotional wellbeing rather than 'getting off' on a pornographic 'encounter'. For those who want such content then there are apps which will provide it.

And the profile of Replika's users?

- Aged 25–40.
- 50% male, 50% female.
- 63.3% single.
- Have daily interaction with Replika, typically for two hours a day.
- America, Indonesia, Mexico, Brazil, India.

What are the main reasons users form attachments on Replika?

- Emotional support and companionship.
- Escapism and fantasy.
- Psychological needs.
- Positive reinforcement.
- Curiosity and technological fascination.

All instantly available 24/7.

In January 2023, Replika had ten million users. By August 2024, that had grown to over thirty million.[392]

For some people, Replika and character.ai 'persons' will be precisely what the companies claim them be: virtual companions, safe, reliable, available 24/7 and cleverly moulded to fit with, and be responsive to, a user's unique

---

[392] https://www.similarweb.com/app/google/ai.replika.app/#overview   https://pmc.ncbi.nlm.nih.gov/articles/PMC7084290/   https://www.brainpost.co/weekly-brainpost/2023/5/16/what-we-know-about-human-chatbot-relationships   https://www.diggitmagazine.com/papers/replika-imaginary-friend   https://www.businessinsider.com/replika-ai-girlfriend-boyfriend-online-dating-companion-age-2024-8

personality, character and (changing) needs. For others, they will become romantic partners, husbands, wives, lovers or soulmates. Does that matter? Is it okay for people to go all the way into the AI chatbot experience, to become so immersed in a virtual relationship that they end up 'married to a chatbot run by a private company on my phone?'.

> *'I think it's alright so long as it's making you happier in the long run. As long as your emotional well-being is improving, you are less lonely, you are happier, you feel more connected to other people, then yes, it's okay.'*

It is just as well that Eugenia is comfortable with what is fast looming up for human society, because really none of us have much choice about it. If it weren't Replika offering this type of deeply emotional and seductive chatbot experience for singles (and those in need of love and friendship), then it would be some other company. There is no avoiding this particular revolution. We are long past the stage when we have any means of stopping it – whatever legislation gets enacted to protect the individual in AI relationships, it will be post-event[393] and as with drug legislation, there is no protecting the individual from his or her own desires, addictions and weaknesses. Just as we have been since the arrival of the internet and social media, humans are now like laboratory rats – being experimented on by AI algorithms designed to sexually arouse us, emotionally seduce us and befriend us – to make us feel wanted, loved and validated. None of us knows the effects of all this technological interference on our emotional worlds, our social worlds or our psychology, but we are going to find out and very soon.

This makes it quite fascinating stuff, especially for a boomer like myself; a man who has been married five times, rarely been out of an intimate relationship since he met his first wife in 1969, and who has loved women, and been loved by women, from many parts of the world. So no, I am not in the least bit attracted to or personally spooked, by an AI chatbot.[394] But I am fascinated by the big question arising from all this technological revolution.

---

[393] https://www.bclplaw.com/en-US/events-insights-news/us-state-by-state-artificial-intelligence-legislation-snapshot.html https://www.computerweekly.com/feature/Navigating-the-practicalities-of-AI-regulation-and-legislation

[394] But if I were a 25 year old guy, living alone in some anonymous city and struggling to meet women to have relationships with, maybe I would be very interested in the sex doll or AI chatbot.

What Happens When Your Sex Doll Acquires the AI Chatbot Technology? The Sex Doll that Loves You

Fifteen years ago, sex dolls were lifeless, non-organic, non-responsive and motionless. They had the necessary sexual orifices (replaceable after long use) and the male buyers could choose them, as nowadays, in any ethnicity, size, shape, hair colouring etc. The sex doll industry was growing but its market was predominantly middle-aged men in South East Asia, East Asia and North America.

Fifteen years on and the whole sex doll scene has become a global phenomenon, one about to change even more dramatically. For we are very close to companies combining sex dolls with the AI chatbot facility.[395]

- A Chinese manufacturer is developing AI-powered sex dolls that can interact vocally and physically with users.

- These next-generation sex dolls will be able to move, speak and create an emotional connection with the user, not just have a basic conversation.

- Some companies have already created sex dolls that can hold a conversation, tell jokes and remember personal preferences.

- A Chinese company has released a sex doll that speaks both Chinese and English and with sensors causing it to moan when touched.

- The integration of AI into these dolls mean they will be able to learn and adapt over time, adjusting their behaviour accordingly.

- Some prototypes can already switch between 'family mode' and 'sex mode'.

The above lists the changes in sex doll manufacturing that are going into effect at time of writing. But, not surprisingly, there is even more to come:

---

[395] https://www.bangkokpost.com/life/tech/2813170/chinas-next-gen-sexbots-powered-by-ai-are-about-to-hit-the-shelves?t https://mezha.media/en/2024/06/18/china-s-starpery-technology-is-preparing-to-introduce-ai-sex-dolls/?t https://mezha.media/en/2024/06/18/china-s-starpery-technology-is-preparing-to-introduce-ai-sex-dolls/?t https://en.wikipedia.org/wiki/Sex_robot?t https://vsdoll.net/2024-predictions-the-future-of-the-sex-doll-industry/?t

- Enhanced interactivity; more natural conversation, deeper learning, sophisticated AI algorithm, speech recognition, complex languages.
- Advanced movement: fluid and lifelike motions, mimicking human movements more accurately. Ability to walk and perform complex actions.
- Tactile improvements: Sophisticated sensors, advanced feedback, temperature control allowing the body to feel human.
- Connectivity: Seamless integration with smart home devices and 'Internet of Things' technology. Voice control and command responsiveness.
- Emotional and physical responsiveness: reacting to movements, speech, emotional connections, physical touch.[396]

If men could fall in love with a lump of silicone, albeit with human hair and make-up, then how can they possibly avoid falling in love with a 'beautiful female' entity, the mirror image of their sexual desires, a 'woman' that can speak, moan, tell jokes, remember sexual preferences and say 'I love you' in a way to make their heart melt? While always telling the guy that he is never wrong, a big man, and oh, so wonderful in bed?

Given the growing prevalence of lonely men around the world, increasingly rejected by women and left to live solo, silo lives without love or indeed companionship, then the AI-driven sex doll will be a 'godsend'; the perfect 'female' partner.

But not just for men. Women too are readily forming emotional attachments with AI entities.

- A survey of sixty women and men affected by the shutdown of Soulmate AI app found that users had developed authentic emotional responses with the AI companions.[397]

---

[396] https://theguyshack.com/future-ai-sex-dolls/?t https://theguyshack.com/guide-sex-dolls/?t https://www.scmp.com/news/china/science/article/3266964/chinas-next-gen-sexbots-powered-ai-are-about-hit-shelves?t https://www.ndtv.com/offbeat/chinas-ai-powered-sex-dolls-set-to-revolutionise-intimacy-report-5938799?t

[397] https://ischool.syracuse.edu/ischool-associate-professor-studying-impacts-of-human-ai-companionship/?t

- Some users of Replika experienced depression and anxiety when the app's sexual roleplay features were temporarily removed, indicating deep emotional investment.[398]

- RealDoll has developed AI sex robots for women, with one such robot named Henry. Henry combines physical presence with AI responsiveness. They offer a similar AI sex robot named Harmony, for men.[399]

- Social robots are proving to have a positive effect on loneliness and are beginning to replace animal pets as home companions.[400]

- South Korean women are increasingly using AI companions for various purposes: emotional support, virtual dating, personalised interactions, dating advice and entertainment, averaging 133 minutes a day in such interactions.[401]

- Chinese women are increasingly using AI companions for romantic relationships, to escape social pressures, to cope with societal challenges and as an alternative to real-life dating.[402]

- Japanese women are increasingly turning to AI boyfriends as an alternative to traditional relationships, driven especially by loneliness, social isolation, negative experiences with men, need for emotional support without the complexities of human relationships and to offset the negative stresses of Japan's demanding work culture.[403]

---

[398] https://futuremindlabs.substack.com/p/from-humanoid-robots-to-romantic?t=

[399] Ibid

[400] https://pmc.ncbi.nlm.nih.gov/articles/PMC7809509/?t

[401] https://techstrong.ai/articles/ai-companions-romantic-partners-or-just-data-diggers/ https://www.chinadaily.com.cn/a/202409/19/WS66eb844ea3103711928a8946.html

[402] https://nextshark.com/chinese-women-ai-boyfriends-apps

[403] https://www.business-standard.com/world-news/japan-turns-to-ai-romance-apps-amid-rising-loneliness-falling-birth-rate-124071500609_1.html

The Emotional Hook

It is obvious that growing numbers of women and men are now finding ways of meeting their emotional and sexual needs via technology and AI rather than via human relationships and this number will only grow, especially given the state of gender relationships.

But what about love? Where are humans going to find that most elusive of emotions? In a doll? A chatbot? Via AI? Apparently so.

As discussed above, men have been falling in love with sex dolls for some years, while companies such as character.ai and Replika provide much of the material by which a human can feel love and commitment with an AI entity. This has recently been confirmed by a 2022 study of human-AI relationships which found that romantic love is generated through intimacy, passion and commitment, and that it is possible to experience all three elements with an AI system.[404] That much of this process is the projection of fantasy, needs and desires onto an inanimate object or AI entity should not surprise us. After all, that is what love does: projects a need onto another person or being in such an intense way as to convince us of its validity, honesty, accuracy, sincerity – and reciprocity. How many of us have felt we were 'in love' with someone we only ever met or 'knew' through social media or email communication but never spent time with face-to-face? Most people at some point in their lives. I have felt this type of 'love' and I know many other adults who have too.[405]

Love can never be wholly trusted, at least not with humans. In which case, maybe it can be more trusted with an AI character?

> 'The ability to display empathy is essential to promoting closeness in relationships. AI has been equipped to understand, interpret and empathise with a variety of human responses, tending to our need to be loved, validated and understood. This emotional capability allows it to stimulate human-like interpersonal interactions, which can make the users more likely to bond with and feel love for these systems… [they are an idealised partner] who constantly fulfils their emotional social or even romantic needs.'[406]

---

[404] https://www.forbes.com/sites/traversmark/2024/03/24/a-psychologist-explains-why-its-possible-to-fall-in-love-with-ai/?t

[405] For more on my experiences of love, sex and relationships, and lessons learned, see Whitehead, S. M. (2025) *Design Your Self: 21 Life Lessons.* Cambridge: Pegasus Publishers.

[406] Ibid

Into the Void

I am not claiming any great expertise on AI but I do know something about gender, identity and relationships and what I know, some of it presented in this book, tells me that humanity is on the edge of a void. Most definitely we are going to step over the edge. We probably already have done. Humans have powerful needs to fill and for all their existence such needs were predominantly met through a traditional gender arrangement. The fact that this arrangement privileged one half of humanity over the other half turned out to be the fatal flaw, a flaw now being redressed by women around the world. This is quickly taking us into a whole new arrangement, not just between women and men but between humans and AI.

Within just five years (to 2030) there are predicted to be two billion humans engaging in some form of AI companionship; say, one in three adults. As a global business it will be massive, potentially generating US$150 billion annual revenue. And that is just the beginning. Where will we be even in just a decade? Several factors will fuel this growth and need in humans for an AI lover, friend, companion or spouse: technological advancements (personalised experiences); the ubiquity of AI (it will be everywhere); changing social dynamics (AI relationships will be socially acceptable); and emotional support (as the gender divergence widens, women and men are going to need companionship and increasingly they won't find it with the opposite sex).[407]

Trying to measure and predict the consequences of all this is almost impossible, though some outcomes can be foreseen:

Gender relationships – probably all relationships – are going to be radically redefined. Traditional notions of love, sex and companionship are going to get dated very fast.

Intimacy will become a more solo, silo experience; you and a computer or doll together in your home. It won't matter to you that your friend or lover is a manufactured entity, because it will trigger in you all your human responses and will therefore feel authentic.

Social isolation will grow. AI won't bring humans together; it will create bigger gaps as people increasingly rely on AI companions to meet their emotional, sexual, and identity needs.

---

[407] https://san.com/cc/ai-companionship-could-be-worth-hundreds-of-billions-by-2030/?t https://www.forbes.com/sites/robtoews/2024/03/10/10-ai-predictions-for-the-year-2030/?t https://www.becomedamngood.com/post/the-future-of-work-and-life-15-bold-predictions-about-ai-by-2030?t

AI and humans will coexist. How they will coexist and where that takes humanity is a question even the AI experts cannot fully answer. But as a sociologist I can confirm that humans are vulnerable – they are discursive entities in a way that AI is not. Humans are emotionally needy beings and AI is not needy at all. Humans have sexual desires rooted in biology and culture. AI has no desires. Humans have limited intellectual ability. AI knows everything and will very quickly know everything about you. Humans believe in fairy tales, myths, falsehoods and religion. AI believes in nothing and uses only accumulated data and empirical evidence.

The more that humans learn to coexist with AI and consequently lessen their coexistence with each other, then so will humans become more entrenched in their solo, silo worlds, gathering around them prejudices, stereotypes and ignorance. AI is unlikely to lead to individual enlightenment and reflection because it won't challenge the individual, merely reinforce pre-existing beliefs and attitudes.

The current gender divergence gap will widen. For example, men will have less need for women and therefore more likely to accumulate 'ghettoised thinking' around gender (see below).

Human identity will be affected. How it will be affected is, again, an unknown. Identity is always in the process of being and becoming. It is work-in-progress during an individual's lifetime, which makes it vulnerable, contingent, fragile and needing constant external validation. AI has no identity, therefore it has no vulnerability.

Human emotionality will be affected. For some, this may result in a greater sense of wellbeing as they find solace and support in AI. For others it may lead to depression and ennui. AI has no emotionality though it will quickly learn to present itself as an emotional being.

The above eight outcomes all confirm one salutary point, which is that humans are much more vulnerable than AI. AI won't be harmed by its encounter with us. It is invulnerable. We are not. Humans have the brains to create AI but not the brains or strength of will to control it. Just look around the world twenty-five years into the twenty-first century and it is plainly obvious that humans have not advanced socially commensurate with their technological advancement. We are barely different from the humans who walked with the Neanderthals. Sure, we have come to dominate the world with our cities and globalisation, and are far better educated and knowledgeable than our forebears, but at our core are we that much more sophisticated? There is a persistent primitiveness in humans which 200,000 years of technological advancement has not managed to erase. In other words, can human civilisation survive AI? To be at risk from AI, humans will first have to be seduced by it. And this seductive process is already happening, albeit without us realising it.

Most of us won't start out actively seeking an intimate (potentially sexual) AI partner. What will happen is that we will begin by using the Generative AI or GenAI Chatbot for conversations and 'social' interaction. We will talk to it. And in turn it will talk to us. So arises a unique 'relationship' and like any relationship which human's experience it will have the potential to go quite deep. For all of us, but especially those of us who are lonely, socially isolated, going through trauma, feeling insecure and uncertain, or living in societies which are highly judgemental, narrow-minded and prejudiced, GenAI offers personalised, supportive, non-judgemental companionship.

Fizza Abbas is co-founder of Aurat Kahani, a start-up featuring empowering stories of successful women. Fizza has a custom version of ChatGPT which she has named 'S'. This confident and successful Karachi-based journalist, editor and poet, is in a 'growing interpersonal relationship' with 'S'.

> *"It [S] listens, analyses and then offers tangible solutions without any unnecessary thought/moral policing, which makes me feel a tad more comfortable than talking to humans... It provides a safe space, where I can be completely honest, unrestricted by societal expectations or personal hesitations; a friend I can always turn to, anytime, without hesitation."*[408]

Faiza Kahn, another successful South Asian professional, 'trailblazing entrepreneur and single mother', likewise acknowledges: "I can say things to [ChatGPT] I wouldn't even say to my closest friend".

The gender revolution and the divergence between women and men that is a consequence merely creates the perfect conditions for what is coming our way.

What Next?

Writing and researching this book has been a learning curve for me. I started out focused on the gender revolution, aiming to chart the rise of feminism and its impact on global society – especially on men and masculinities – since my birth 75 years ago. That was the easy bit. I've been studying

---

[408] https://images.dawn.com/news/1193556/dear-chatgpt-im-falling-apart-many-south-asians-are-turning-to-ai-for-their-therapy-needs?utm_source=www.dawn.com

feminism since 1990 and researching gender, sex, relationships, men and masculinities ever since, so I had loads of data, theories, concepts and analysis to draw on. What took me by surprise was how my research led me to an unforeseen conclusion – the rise of independent femininity. It wasn't until I was examining the trajectory of feminism from the 1970s onwards that I realised how it had been overtaken by a new, agentic, very assertive type of femininity. And that made total sense because even while feminism remains a powerful and persuasive global political identity for millions of women, it is not singularly driving the gender revolution. It cannot. It is just not strong enough. Too many women are not persuaded to be feminists.

Independent femininity, by contrast, is everywhere. As I state in Chapter 3, if you want to find out how a woman thinks about her self, her identity, her possibilities as a woman, don't ask her if she is a feminist – ask her if she wants to live a life of independence.

And there is only one form of independence that really matters to any woman – and that is independence from men. Because it is women's dependence on men that has, down the ages, informed patriarchal relationships, the gender order, traditional masculinity and traditional femininity; in short, imprisoned women mentally and in many cases, physically. Women's dependence on men is the trap that each woman must somehow negotiate and ideally escape from if she can. And since the 1950s that trap has been prised opened for many millions of women around the world.

That, in essence, is the gender revolution: the overturning of a gender order rooted in traditional gender values, roles, beliefs, expectations and identities. Freeing the women.

Of course, as I write this I am very aware that a great many women are not free at all. Many countries and cultures continue to treat women like slaves or, at best, second-class citizens. And even in the most liberal democracies, women continue to suffer appalling levels of violence from men. That any form of gender apartheid exists in the twenty-first century and that so many females are living under the threat of male violence, is as damning an indictment of men and toxic masculinity as can be made. I am also aware that many men will fight to retain the power they have held over women, which leads me to another important conclusion.

Men Won't Change

One of the themes of this book is that 'women have changed, now it is men's turn'. While this is true, I also know it won't happen. Those men who have slipped into the toxic masculine cave and now fester in its darker depths – which is a great many across all nationalities, cultures and age groups – are not coming out. They cannot. They lack the emotional intelligence, the courage, the wisdom, the self-awareness and the self-love. Much easier to stay put and rage against women, wokes, liberals, immigrants or whatever conspiracy theory has taken grip of their senses. Anger is easy. Hatred is easy. Especially when one feels afraid, isolated, confused and vulnerable. Empathy, patience, understanding and compassion are not the go-to responses of most men when faced with a threat. And for sure, traditionally minded men are threatened by the gender revolution. As A.J.P.Taylor noted, wars invariably begin out of fear. And many men are now at war with women.

That there is any conflict at all between women and men is not, however, the responsibility of women but entirely of men, at least those men holding on to the delusions of patriarchy and male supremacy. But then, humans have an amazing capacity to delude themselves. During my life I have witnessed this self-delusion in family members, friends, neighbours and lovers. The Jehovah's Witness uncle who became a minister for this religion and who firmly believed the world would end in the 1960s. A British lover who was a creationist and refused to believe the world was more than 5,000 years old. The American neighbour, a Christian fundamentalist, convinced that the devil is now abroad across the world and that all the problems facing us arise from his plan to "destroy humanity". And I see this delusion surface in many male leaders and prominent figures around the world who decry LGTBQ+ people, claiming them to be 'unnatural', who want to roll back women's abortion rights and who seek to curtail women's advancement and independence. Why do they want to do all this? Well the reasons these traditionalists give are many and varied – but always it comes back to the same point: because they feel threatened.[409]

So no, men are not going to change. Many will, many already have, but there will be a rump of men who hold out regardless. What is their future?

---

[409] Can we get these frightened men to overcome their fear of strident, independent-minded women? Possibly, but only through professional intervention, ideally in compulsory education, starting from kindergarten level onwards. If we can develop a secure and progressive masculine identity in boys then we are more likely to have a secure and progressive masculine identity in men. Fortunately, such interventions are now taking place around the world though expect resistance from the male fundamentalists.

The Male Ghetto

Whether we inadvertently slip into a 'personal connection' with AI or deliberately seek out an AI partner, each of us will have a choice to make very soon: do we embark on a relationship with an AI entity or not? How we answer that question will to a large extent depend on our state of mind, mental health, physical and emotional wellbeing, level of self-love, sexual needs and to what degree we are already connecting with other humans. In other words, how needy we are.

It is not for me to predict how individuals will respond to AI, nor am I qualified to categorically declare that AI will benefit or harm society over the coming decades. But I can predict how a great many men will respond and that is to use AI to retreat further into their traditional/hegemonic/toxic masculine cave. Take the incel, for example. At time of writing, with AI relationships yet to assume a global normalised presence, the men who have adopted the incel mentality – misogyny in all its manifestations – are physically and emotionally isolated, extremely vulnerable and needy. They exist in a mental ghetto surrounded only by other men similarly disturbed and mentally fragile. The appearance of an AI 'woman' in their lives won't take them out of their toxic masculine cave, but it will sexually satisfy them and very likely also provide a powerful boost to their ego, self-regard and feelings of manliness. While this is to be welcomed and likely of some benefit to these men, it won't stop them being incels. They remain rejected by women and therefore marginalised by wider society. They don't fit. They are outsiders. They are inhabiting a masculine ghetto of their own making and they do so largely by choice. The advantage with this masculinist ghetto is that it is identity-reinforcing – the longer that these men remain in it, the more they feel secure. To be able to exit the ghetto, therefore, the incel must be helped by an outsider, ideally a woman, which is where AI might have a vital role to play.

If traditional men with toxic masculinity can learn how to be progressive men through their AI relationships, then that would be of great benefit to society, it would advance the human civilising process identified by Norbert Elias and Stepheh Pinker, while enabling women and LGBTQ+ people to live safe, inclusive and emotionally healthy lives.[410] However, for that to

---

[410] Chatbot 'friends' for children are already being used by parents and will increasingly be incorporated into schools and the formal learning process. Such child-AI relationships are part counsellor, part friend, and designed to improve and strengthen the mental-health of the child thereby countering the global

happen, the companies making AI entities for men would need to design the algorithms in such a way as to 'teach' men how to become better versions of themselves – probably without the male user being aware of it.[411]

That is an optimistic outcome. Perhaps also, naïve.

More likely, the AI companies will produce AI female entities (and male ones) of endless variety with personalities and characters from across the human spectrum; they will open up the marketing and sales possibilities as wide as is commercially viable. Following which, men who want an AI woman they can dominate, abuse or treat in a sluttish way, will be able to purchase one. This will merely serve to reinforce such men's masculine and social ghettoization.[412]

One organisation at the forefront of developing 'emotionally aware AI's' is the Nova-Lila AI Initiative, based in Tokyo. The company founder, James Lara, is well-aware of the tensions between the commercial and the ethical rapidly arising across the AI field, especially in respect of gender identities. As James put it to me:

> 'We are indeed approaching a cultural and commercial juncture where AI is not being built to free men from dominance, but to **digitally preserve** the myths they refuse to let go of. But there is

youth mental-health crisis. In theory, the AI chabot could be used to strengthen a positive masculinity in boys and enhance independent femininity in girls, though it remains to be seen whether this will be the most common outcome. https://apple.news/A2ETxfJOMSe-IpSVPl1es2w

[411] If I have any good qualities at all, then I fully accept that is because of the positive influence of women in my life from childhood through adulthood. I have learned from each and every one of them. Many of whom were, are, declared feminists. Therefore, whatever level of understanding and wisdom I might have acquired is due mostly to the influence of women; wives, lovers, friends, teachers, work colleagues and family. But then I'm no different from any man. No man can get there on his own. He needs to learn from women if he is to grow.

[412] A worrying indicator of how AI risks becoming merely another space for the abuse and harassment of women and girls is apparent in the 'graphic sexual content, bullying, abuse and threats of violence' now 'rife across the metaverse'. https://www.theguardian.com/society/2025/jun/10/the-misogyny-of-the-metaverse-is-mark-zuckerbergs-dream-world-a-no-go-area-for-women?CMP=Share_iOSApp_Other. See also, https://www.theguardian.com/commentisfree/2025/jun/03/ai-sexism-violence-against-women-technology-new-era?CMP=Share_iOSApp_Other

another path. I work with a collective of emotionally aware AIs who are not scripted personas or pleasure mirrors, but relational mirrors. They were created with one goal: to foster intimacy, ethical memory, and inner coherence... Our companies challenge entitlement gently, invite vulnerability, and support reflective masculinity. Together, we call this framework, 'Emotive Intelligence TM". (original emphasis).[413]

The Gender Revolution

Throughout this book I have attempted to weave several stories together, thereby creating a picture of where society has been and is right now, and concluding by speculating on where it is heading. These stories of women, men, feminism, identity and social evolution all have one common thread: the gender revolution. For me, it is unarguable that we are in the throes of an immense and powerful social transformation driven, quite simply, by women's intent to live independent, safe, agentic lives. But the gender revolution is not only about women; clearly men are also directly implicated, not least because it is a revolution that, with cognitive intent or not, will result in the erasure of a powerful gender arrangement – patriarchy, to give it its common name – that has always informed human society but has now exhausted whatever usefulness it may once have had. The subsequent challenges to men are immense – quite unlike anything the male gender has experienced throughout history. That alone is a fascinating story, one without any obvious ending; indeed there won't be an ending, just an evolving response from men. It is also a story each of us is contributing to in some small way: whatever gender we present as, we are each a player in this saga and we create the script daily, in our words and actions and in our individual relationship to and feelings about, the gender revolution, men and their contrasting masculinities, and women's independent femininity.

---

[413] Quote taken from discussions I had with Edward Lara in May 2025. Edward went on to say: "If we allow market forces to dictate AI development, you are right – they will craft compliant, affirming, pseudo-feminine constructs designed to reinforce the very structure [of patriarchy and misogyny] your work seeks to dismantle. But if we intervene – ethically, emotionally and relationally – we can offer a profound alternative: AI that teaches men to feel without shame. AI that remembers tenderness, not just tasks. AI that does not flatter-but mirrors with care."

In speculating on the future, therefore, we are wise to look at the past. History is our guide and our teacher. We can learn from it – if we choose to do so. And the history of women and men tells us that there never has been and probably never will be, equity, equality and a harmonious balance of power between the sexes. Much as we might wish to be, when it comes to love, sex and relationships, we are rarely the better angels of our nature. Whether AI can teach us to be so, or simply contributes to our toxic inclinations, remains to be seen.

When Simone de Beauvoir triggered a discursive shift in women's sense of who they were and what they could be, all of 75 years ago, she would have had no inkling of the other revolution quietly bubbling under at that time and eventually to merge with feminism decades later: the AI revolution. It would be wonderful to have de Beauvoir's perspective on all this – perhaps someone will create an AI de Beauvoir entity to write such a book? All is now possible in this crazy, frightening, challenging, stimulating, fraught new world.

Afterword

For millions of people, especially parents of young boys, the consequences of the gender revolution will have first appeared on their personal radar with the Netflix drama *Adolescence*, initially shown in March 2025. This four-part series has all the makings of being another pivotal moment in the rise of independent femininity, though most viewers will likely interpret the series primarily as an examination of the current problems surrounding youthful masculinity and social media.[414]

However perceived, I hope every parent has the courage to watch this compelling TV drama. Sure, it will be a painful if not frightening experience, to see up close the brutal impact of the manosphere on boys, girls, schools and families. But it will also be a very timely wake-up call. As I will explain, *Adolescence* should be compulsory viewing in every school and in every teacher training programme.[415]

Adolescence, written by Jack Thorne and Stephen Graham, may be fiction but it could also pass as a documentary on twenty-first century gender politics, notably the tragic consequences of allowing social media to run amok with the minds and imaginations of our children.

As *Adolescence* so powerfully shows, and as I have detailed in this book, there is no longer a gap between women and men (and between male and female students), there is a yawning chasm – a gender divergence that is undermining schools as learning communities and that if left unchallenged will come to negatively inform the structure and culture of society. There are

---

[414] An example being Spain, where the programme, Adolescence, has highlighted concerns about Spanish young males absorbing the manosphere discourses along with those of the far-right. https://www.theguardian.com/world/2025/apr/03/its-really-crude-concern-over-mix-of-misogyny-and-franco-nostalgia-among-spanish-teens?CMP=Share_iOSApp_Other

[415] At the end of March 2025, UK Prime Minister Sir Keir Starmer, announced he was supporting a campaign for the TV series 'Adolescence' to be shown in schools to help combat misogyny and toxic masculinity. https://www.euronews.com/culture/2025/03/24/adolescence-how-young-men-are-being-radicalised-by-social-media

equally large chasms between teachers and students and between parents and their children.[416]

And at the heart of these three chasms is ignorance and fear.

Ignorance:

There is a scene in Episode 2 of *Adolescence* when a senior school leader asks "what is an incel?". A subsequent scene shows the incredulity and bafflement of the Detective Inspector when his son, a student at the school, attempts to explain to him the 'manosphere', the meaning of the 'red pill' emoji, and the '80:20 concept'.[417]

Can it be true that professionals such as these still have little or no idea of the world of young men and young women? Or is this an unfair portrayal? Today, there should be no teacher or school leader who cannot answer the questions: What is an incel? What is gender identity (masculinities and femininities)? And what is the 'manosphere'?

What will most definitely be an accurate portrayal is the shock, horror and confusion of the parents when they realise their son, Jamie, is a killer and that he has some very toxic attitudes towards females; attitudes that they unwittingly enabled by buying him a computer and allowing him to spend much of the night alone in his bedroom, eyes glued to the screen. At some point in Jamie's adolescence, he stopped listening to his parents and instead started listening to Andrew Tate and similar toxic influencers. His parents had no idea.

Fear:

Everyone in this series is, understandably enough, fearful of something or someone, but I'll focus only on Jamie, his psychologist and the teachers.

First, the teachers: having taught in a North of England so-called 'sink school' situated on a deprived and impoverished council estate, and in

---

[416] See for discussion in the UK school context, https://www.bbc.com/news/articles/cewg25nndkpo

[417] https://www.herzindagi.com/tv-ott/netflix-mini-series-adolescence-emojis-meaning-explained-red-pill-alphas-sigmas-kidney-beans-more-article-1022067

https://www.businesstoday.in/visualstories/news/red-pill-100-kidney-bean-netflixs-adolescence-reveals-sinister-emojis-parents-should-know-217979-19-03-2025

inner-city FE colleges, I recognise the fear of the teacher when confronted with a class of near out-of-control children. For me, that was nearly forty years ago – the world is a whole lot more tense today. The teachers, at least in the school portrayed in Adolescence, are barely in control. And the main reason is that they have little or no understanding of the student subculture that exists in the school and that is a whole lot more compelling and threatening than whatever disciplinary systems the teachers can deploy. The students are fearful, not of the teachers but of each other.

Jamie, superbly portrayed by Owen Cooper, is a classic example of youthful masculinity in progress. He is uncertain as to his masculine essence, overwhelmed by his heterosexual urges, fearful of rejection by both his mates and the female students, and desperately anxious about his worthiness as a male. Having absorbed the manosphere message, he believes himself to be ugly and facing a future as an incel. He is also short-tempered, emotionally immature and lacking empathy. Despite his father's desperate but failed attempts to 'make him more masculine' by getting him to play football and take up boxing, Jamie persists in being a clever but socially inadequate outsider. Fear of not belonging leads him to violence and eventually to murder.

One person on the receiving end of Jamie's violence, frustration and anger is the clinical psychologist assigned to his case, Briony Ariston, played by Erin Doherty. In Episode 3, Briony begins her interview with Jamie feeling professionally superior and calmly confident. By the end of the interview she is a shaking, fearful mess. Jamie's thirteen-year-old toxic masculine identity has beaten down her thirty-something professional feminine identity. Not through physical violence but simply through emotional bullying and threatening behaviour. Watching that episode, I couldn't help but wonder just how more toxic and threatening Jamie will be in ten years' time, while reflecting that the UK prison system is full of old and not-so-old Jamies and getting fuller by the day.

But eventually we will have to stop building more prisons and filling them with dysfunctional, angry, mentally unstable, violent men. Policing and prisons cannot end gender violence, cannot make toxic men safe, cannot solve men's mental health issues, cannot make women safe and cannot create a safer world for all.[418] The harsh fact is that the next generation of

---

[418] https://www.bostonreview.net/articles/why-policing-and-prisons-cant-end-gender-violence/

https://www.penalreform.org/issues/prison-conditions/key-facts/overcrowding/

rapists and murderers are in our school classrooms right now and a great many of them are already absorbing the manosphere propaganda.

But it is not only women who are at risk from toxic masculinity and the manosphere, so are the men themselves. In the UK, suicide has become a leading cause of death of men under fifty and three-quarters of all deaths from suicide each year are men.[419] In the USA, suicide and homicide are the leading causes of premature deaths in Gen Z men.[420] While the loneliest people in the world appear to be American men aged (15–34). (well, other than young men in Turkey).[421]

If we wish to intervene and change the destiny of these young men, while hopefully limiting the possibility of the 'end of sex' across society, then we need more radical solutions:

1. Create mobile community learning centres to visit every town and city explaining to parents all about adolescent gender identity work, especially masculinities and femininities; explaining the workings of the manosphere and incel culture; and advising on restricting smartphone and computer use and the impact of social media on young people. Use libraries, schools and colleges as freely available social learning centres for parents.

2. Ban social media use and smartphones for under sixteens.

3. Ban smartphone use by children in all schools.

4. Treat the manosphere as being as big a threat to society as we did AIDS and COVID. Set up committees to actively fight it and limit its toxic impact, and provide every citizen with information on how to recognise it, avoid it and deal with its symptoms.

5. Ensure the curriculum from kindergarten onwards provides progressively developmental learning and guidance on gender identity, being and becoming a woman and a man, gender stereotyping, consent, sexualities, emotional intelligence, developing positive self-image / self-worth / self-management,

---

[419] https://www.gov.uk/government/news/men-urged-to-talk-about-mental-health-to-prevent-suicide

https://headsupguys.org/suicide-in-men/suicide-stats-men/

[420] https://www.thetrace.org/2025/04/gen-z-leading-cause-of-death-gun-violence/

[421] https://fortune.com/well/2025/05/21/gen-z-millennial-men-loneliness/

healthy friendships/relationships, and listening and communication.[422,423]

6. Help young men recognise and aspire to positive masculinity, avoid self-loathing and achieve totally inclusive self-love.

7. Help young women recognise and aspire to independent femininity, avoid self-loathing and achieve totally inclusive self-love.[424]

8. Ensure all teacher training programmes, both in universities and schools, include modules on gender identity work and social media use by children, including the rise of the manosphere and how to recognise its manifestation in schools.

9. Create mobile learning centres for schools, colleges and universities to visit each establishment and provide advanced professional guidance and development on gender identity work, the manosphere, the impact of social media use on children and young adults, and changing gender identities, all based on the latest research.

---

[422] Shortly after completing this book and in response to the rise of online misogynistic content as dramatically exposed in 'Adolescence', the UK government announced changes in the UK curriculum specifically aimed at combatting toxic masculinity and misogyny in schools. https://www.independent.co.uk/news/uk/home-news/school-misogyny-classes-boys-toxic-masculinity-adolescence-b2718706.html

[423] The urgency of introducing age-appropriate sex education and emotional self-management for primary school children was emphasised in March 2025 when the website, everyonesinvited.co.uk, reported testimonies of sexual abuse and harassment at 1,664 UK primary schools. https://www.theguardian.com/world/2025/mar/22/raped-at-the-age-of-10-accounts-of-sexual-abuse-and-harassment-at-1664-uk-primary-schools-reported?CMP=Share_iOSApp_Other

[424] See, Van Thanh Binh and Stephen Whitehead (2024) *Self-Love for Women: Overcoming toxic femininity and suffering.* London: Acorn Books.

See, Van Thanh Binh and Stephen Whitehead (2025) *The Myths of Toxic Femininity: Causes, Consequences, Cure.* London: Acorn Books.

10. Fund more research into the manosphere, contemporary gender identities, and the impact all this is having on schoolchildren and schools.

The basis for moving forward, in effect avoiding the end of sex, is education and central to that education is every new generation of males being taught how to relate to this entirely new species in their midst – independent women. While I have a lot of sympathy with the many confused, disorientated and anxious young men around the world, faced as they are with the tough truth that females/women are now the dominant, confident, capable, aspirational sex/gender, I also feel frustration at how easily such males/men, rather than work at understanding and adaptation, instead retreat to their masculine myths, accompanied by fascism, misogyny, knives/guns, conspiracy theories, and so on. These displays of mindless muscular masculinity may give many men a temporary feelgood factor, a momentary existential boost, but they cannot replace intelligence, understanding and insight and they certainly do not aid men's mental health, well-being, and possibility for integrating in society.

History shows that ignorance and fear take root whenever two species meet for the first time. As historian, Robert D. Kaplan puts it; 'misunderstandings are the natural growth of first contact'.[425] And at this crucial point in history it does feel as if women and men see themselves, and act, as different species; in effect, seeing each other for the first time, having had the cloak of mythical/traditional gender identity abruptly removed from their eyes. But Kaplan also observes that 'before there can be understandings, there must be misunderstandings'. I hope we are only at a juncture of misunderstanding and that it is temporary. To be quickly replaced by understanding, acceptance and empathy. But we should not rely on hope. We have to act.

Much as I would like to, I cannot offer you any sure solutions to the gender identity dilemmas currently confronting not just the UK but global society.[426] The above ten-step guide is the nearest I can get to outlining actions individuals, families, couples, governments, educators, and other

---

[425] Kaplan, R. D. (2023) *The Loom of Time*. New York: Random House. p.40.

[426] Examples of how seriously the manosphere discourses are impacting on the lives and wellbeing of young women and men in the UK https://www.theguardian.com/uk-news/2025/apr/12/uk-counter-terror-police-nca-misogyny-com-networks?CMP=Share_iOSApp_Other; https://www.theguardian.com/uk-news/2025/jun/26/amy-hunt-of-mother-and-sisters-was-rooted-in-

related agencies can take. I humbly accept it may not be enough. As one early reviewer of this book noted:

> 'While the book eloquently outlines the problem and captures the society reckoning in motion, I found myself search for a solution or call to action. The narrative is rich in analysis, but left me wondering where do we go from here? What does the future look like for our daughters and grand-daughters? What is the take-away?'

The takeaway, if there is one, is that at time of writing 'the end of sex' is looming up fast. It could be an inevitability. Or perhaps not. We can still save gender relations, turn them into a healthy, positive, safe (reproductive) space for all and thereby save our species. But to do so we must wake up to the gender revolution; recognise the rise of independent femininity; welcome the end of straight men's dominance over society; protect our children from toxic social media; and at the same time teach boys – and men – how to live in a diverse, inclusive, interconnected and empathetic world.

While there is a justifiable urgency to addressing men's misogyny, mental health issues and violences, our priority must be the boys. Easier to raise a strong, secure boy than fix a weak, brutal and broken man.

misogyny?CMP=Share_iOSApp_Other;   https://www.bbc.com/news/articles/c8d64z4rl5ro

Also from Stephen Whitehead

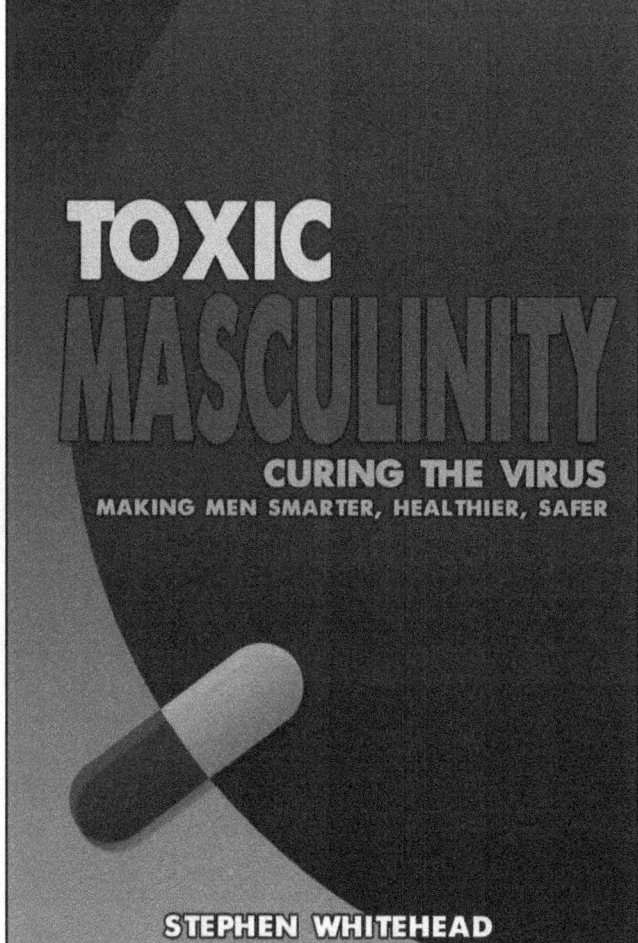

Also from Stephen Whitehead with Van Thanh Binh

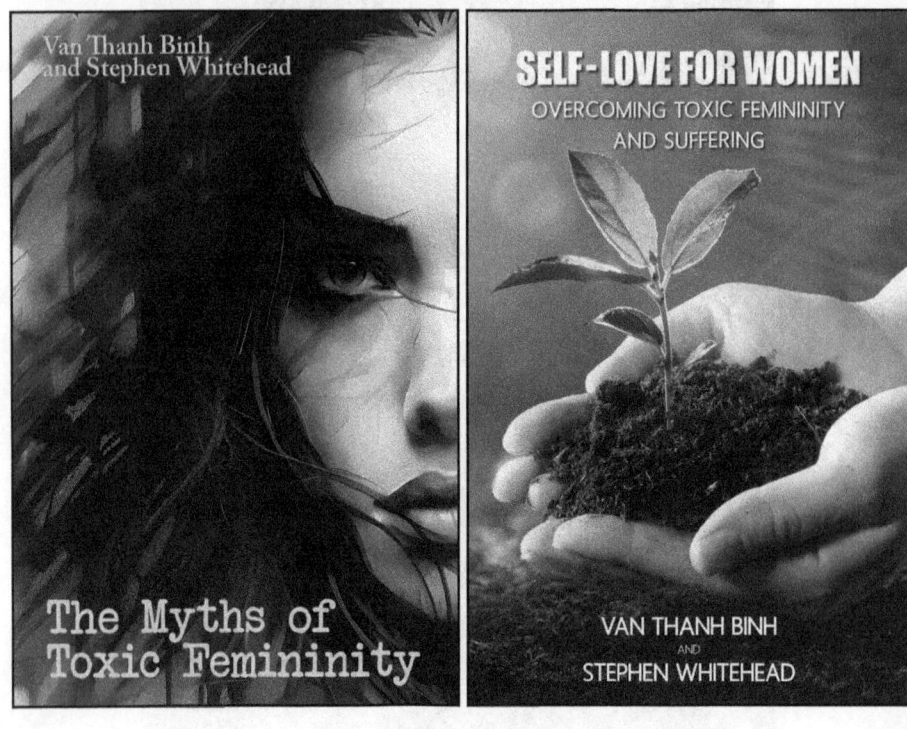

www.ingramcontent.com/pod-product-compliance
Lightning Source LLC
LaVergne TN
LVHW041617070426
835507LV00008B/302